**The Johns Hopkins Series in
Contemporary Medicine and Public Health**

Consulting Editors
Samuel H. Boyer IV, M.D.
Gareth M. Green, M.D.
Richard T. Johnson, M.D.
Paul R. McHugh, M.D.
Edmond A. Murphy, M.D.
Albert H. Owens, Jr., M.D.
Edyth H. Schoenrich, M.D., M.P.H.
Jerry L. Spivak, M.D.
Barbara H. Starfield, M.D., M.P.H.

Automated Blood Counts and Differentials

A Practical Guide

J. DAVID BESSMAN, M.D.
Associate Professor of Medicine and Pathology
University of Texas Medical Branch

The Johns Hopkins University Press
Baltimore and London

Second printing, paperback, 1988

The Johns Hopkins University Press
701 West 40th Street
Baltimore, Maryland 21211
The Johns Hopkins Press Ltd., London

Library of Congress Cataloging-in-Publication Data

Bessman, J. David.
  Automated blood counts and differentials.

  (The Johns Hopkins series in contemporary medicine
and public health)
  Bibliography: p.
  Includes index.
  1. Blood cell count—Automation—Handbooks, manuals,
etc. 2. Blood—Examination—Handbooks, manuals, etc.
3. Blood—Diseases—Diagnosis—Handbooks, manuals,
etc. I. Title. II. Series.
RB45.B39 1986   616.07′561   85-24108
ISBN 0-8018-3171-7 (alk. paper)
ISBN 0-8018-3173-3 (pbk. : alk. paper)

To my parents

Contents

Contents

CONTENTS

List of Figures and Tables

Figures

Tables

LIST OF FIGURES AND TABLES

Acknowledgments

It was my privilege to learn from mentors who were not only recognized scientists, but generous teachers. Further, my chiefs—Abraham Goldin, Donald Feinstein, Lockard Conley, and Frank Gardner—provided superb training and the opportunity to develop independently. It is no accident that many successful investigators have emerged at each of their laboratories.

Many colleagues have given valuable and helpful advice. Wendy A. Harris and Mary Lou Kenney, of the Johns Hopkins University Press, were indispensable in turning a hopeful letter into a book. Dr. Alvin Lewis, author of two books, reassured me that it could be done. I am especially grateful for the patience and understanding of my wife, Joan, and our children, Daniel, Elizabeth, and Matthew. They have accepted the intrusions into their time and space and have provided constant encouragement.

I could not have started a career in academic medicine without the example of imagination and intellectual integrity provided by my parents, Drs. Samuel and Alice Bessman. I could not have continued without their love and encouragement.

Introduction

There is a wide gap between the data that medical research and technology make possible and how these data are used. This book addresses this gap in regard to automated blood counts and differentials. It informs the reader not only of the new terminology of automated blood counting but also of how the new data improve diagnostic ability. The new information confirms some unproved concepts and challenges others. This book is not intended to be even a short text of general hematology, but brief descriptions of the physiology underlying blood cell size and heterogeneity are provided throughout the text. When this discussion is speculative, it is identified as such.

Interpreting the variables and histograms of automated hematology and correlating these with manual blood smear morphology will challenge both the technician operating the equipment and the physician receiving the report (Jen et al. 1983; Hanson et al. 1985). The new information will make hematologic diagnosis more rapid and more precise, providing data that cannot be obtained with manual microscopy. This book is designed to make the reader sufficiently familiar with these data that he or she will be able to interpret an automated blood count report with the same skill that is used to interpret an electrocardiogram or chest x-ray. Just as the latter complement manual auscultation of the chest, the automated blood count can comple-

ment manual microscopy. The principles of histogram and slide analysis are presented here in
a manner that applies to all commercial
instruments.

The reader may want to consult an "expert" on
difficult or unusual data, but should be able to
analyze the routine abnormal blood counts (just
as would be the case for the common electrocardiogram or chest x-ray). The self-test examples at the end of the book will help the reader
to reach this goal.

In addition to appropriate references, unpublished data from this laboratory's experience
are included, especially in areas where there is
widespread use of automated data without extensive publication in peer-reviewed journals.

This book is not a comprehensive guide to the
technical details of the automated instruments.
However, it contains the information necessary
to understand the data they provide and the artifacts that occur. For a more thorough technical
discussion, other sources are available (England
1984). The manufacturer's manual often is most
detailed. Unlike the x-ray or electrocardiogram,
both the mechanics and the format of data reported by automated hematological instruments
vary among manufacturers and change from
year to year. To avoid "dating" this book, or
showing inappropriate bias toward a particular
manufacturer, I have presented the individual
case illustrations in a format that does not copy
any commercial instrument's.The data formats of
individual instruments (including some data
under development) at the time of press are
shown in appendix B. The majority of the data
illustrated were obtained on a Coulter Counter
S-Plus IV.

Finally, the data of the automated blood count
alone will not guarantee a specific diagnosis in
every case, nor does every disease have a
single pattern of abnormality. Few laboratory
data can be this specific. Rather, these values

should be used to narrow the differential as much as possible, so that more expensive and time-requiring definitive or confirmatory tests can be done as selectively and rapidly as possible.

**Automated
Blood Counts
and
Differentials**

1

The Automation of Hematology

Until about 1955, quantitative laboratory hematology depended on counting chambers and
manually reviewing stained blood smears. Careful technique allowed a sophisticated analysis of
red cell disorders and a semiqualitative platelet
count and white cell distribution measurement
(Wintrobe 1981; Koepke 1978). In the past thirty
years, there has been a crescendo of improve-
ments to automated techniques.

1955 impedance counters of single cell types
1967 semiautomated red cell and white cell
      counts and red cell indices
1972 automated cytochemistry leukocyte
      differential
1979 automated platelet counts, red cell dis-
      tribution width measurement, and plate-
      let size measurement
1981 automated impedance white cell differ-
      ential and cell size distributions

Two general technologies are used in automated
blood counting today: flow cytometry and image
analysis. Flow cytometry uses a thin, high-speed
jet of diluent fluid in which suspended cells move
in single file past a sensor. The sensor measures the presence or absence of a specified
variable (e.g., impedance, light scatter, or
enzyme content) in each cell as it passes the
sensor (fig. 1.1; at present, commercial instruments use the techniques as displayed in table
1.1). The particular strength of flow cytometry is

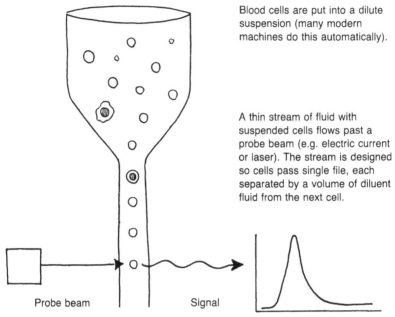

Blood cells are put into a dilute suspension (many modern machines do this automatically).

A thin stream of fluid with suspended cells flows past a probe beam (e.g. electric current or laser). The stream is designed so cells pass single file, each separated by a volume of diluent fluid from the next cell.

Probe beam

Signal

Interaction of the probe beam with the cell causes a signal to be sent. The signal is proportional to the amount of the variable being measured in each individual cell (e.g. size or fluorescence).

Data are collected, typically for 10,000 individual cells. The data are displayed and printed in histogram or scattergram form.

FIGURE 1.1
General scheme of flow cytometry instruments.

its rapidity and the high number of single cells that may be analyzed for several variables simultaneously; also, the cells examined can, as a group, be retrieved in suspension or on a slide for further use. The weakness is that once a cell passes the sensor, it becomes anonymous among other cells processed: a single ambiguous cell cannot be retrieved for positive confirmation.

Image analysis depends on cells fixed on a slide and analyzed by high-speed optics on a special stage, according to programmed criteria. The strength of this technique is that most programs include a memory that will relocate and display exactly those cells requested. The major shortcomings are that about one-tenth as many

TABLE 1.1   Properties of Some Common Automated Blood Counters

Instrument	Platelet Analysis	Red Blood Cell Analysis (RBC)	White Blood Cell Analysis (WBC)
S-Plus Series (Coulter Electronics, Hialeah, Fla.)	Impedance	Impedance	Impedance
H-6000/601 (Technicon, Tarrytown, N.Y.)	Light scatter	Light scatter	Enzyme content and light scatter
ELT-8 (Ortho, Westwood, Mass.)	Light scatter	Light scatter	Light scatter
Sysmex E-5000 (Toa, Del Amo, Calif.)	Impedance	Impedance	Impedance

cells as in flow cytometry can be processed in a similar time, and further use of the cells that are analyzed is limited by slide preparation (van Assendelft and England 1982). Also, image analysis has not been satisfactorily combined with cell counting. Therefore, routine instruments increasingly are of the flow cytometry technology.

Both technologies are much more rapid than manual methods and measure many more cells; this is a marked advance for differential counts of leukocytes. Equally important, cell characteristics that in the past were reported only as a mean can now be displayed to show the distribution among the cells measured—as histograms of a single variable's distribution and scattergrams of two variables' correlate distribution. These data advance automated hematology not only in precision but also in new definitions of normality and new classifications of disease. A mean value may be normal or abnormal, but the distribution of a histogram may be normal or abnormal independent of the mean. Histograms may be described by mean, heterogeneity, and shape. Heterogeneity often is reported as the coefficient of variation, CV, which is standard deviation divided by mean. If the normal histogram is known to have a characteristic shape (approximately Gaussian for red cell and white cell volume, clearly right-skewed for platelet volume), any change from the normal shape can be noted by examination of the histogram. A distribution may have an increased CV caused by two or more distinct populations or by increased variation about a single mean. Examples in the text illustrate this.

Some of the variables that are reported depend on ad hoc assumptions of cellular properties that are made by the instruments' programs. These assumptions are discussed in the appropriate sections.

Although these machines measure hematologic values in terms established by manual microscopy and chamber counting, the actual measurements now are quite different. For example, the classical hematocrit was a measure of packed red cell volume. The automated hematocrit is the product of red cell count times the average red cell size (therefore, not including trapped plasma). The two hematocrits rarely are precisely the same, and when abnormal red cell shape affects the automated cell size or the packing of spun cells (see below), the two hematocrit values will diverge. Other differences are listed in the individual sections.

2
Red Cells

2.1   Introduction: Normal Values

The clinician and the laboratory technologist should know where and how the values given as "normal" ranges have been obtained. Some measures vary by age, such as mean cell volume (MCV) and mean cell hemoglobin (MCH); by sex, such as red blood cell count (RBC), hemoglobin (Hb), and hematocrit (Hct); or by race, white blood cell count (WBC). The range of variation of values among normal subjects should be clear. The technical replicate error for each determination should be known. Our hospital's normal values (table 2.1) are drawn from 1,000 entering students of medicine, nursing, and allied health, aged seventeen to thirty years, and from 580 infants (Bessman and Dover 1979). The replicate error is the range that may be expected among measurements of ten aliquots of the same sample. They differ little from many published lists of normals (Bull and Hay 1985; Williams 1983; Wintrobe 1981), but each laboratory should either have its own reference range or show the source of these reference values.

The variation among normals must be borne in mind when considering abnormalities. For instance, in a normal individual red cell values vary little (essentially only machine error) over time, so it is most useful to judge normality against the subject's own past values (if available) rather than the "normal range." For the

TABLE 2.1 Normal Values for Automated Blood Counts

Item	Mean	±2 SD	Replicate Error
RBC	$5.41 \times 10^{12}/l$*	$0.72 \times 10^{12}/l$	$0.15 \times 10^{12}/l$
Hb	16.1 g/dl*	2.0 g/dl	0.2 g/dl
Hct	48.6%*	5.1%	1.3%
MCV	90.3 fl[†]	9.6 fl	2.4 fl
MCH	29.1 pg	2.1 pg	0.7 pg
MCHC	33.6%	1.8%	1.1%
Platelets	$283 \times 10^{9}/l$	$141 \times 10^{9}/l$	$12 \times 10^{9}/l$
WBC	$6.1 \times 10^{9}/l$[‡]	$2.4 \times 10^{9}/l$	$0.3 \times 10^{9}/l$
RDW	13.2%	1.6%	0.5%

*These values are for white males only. Normal values for females are approximately 12 percent less. For blacks the values are an additional 5 percent less for males or females (Meyers et al. 1979; Castro et al. 1985). Bone marrow reserves decrease during old age (Lipschitz et al. 1981). Among the peripheral-blood values, only RBC, Hb, and Hct decline, by about 10 percent, in normal subjects over 45 years of age (unpublished data).

[†]These values are for adults only. Newborns have increased MCV (101 ± 13) and RDW ($16.8 \pm 1.9\%$). These values fall progressively to a nadir at about 6 months old, with an MCV of 76 ± 10 fl and normal RDW. MCV then slowly rises, reaching normal values in early adulthood. The mean value from 6 months up to age 20 can be approximated as $75 + 0.8$ (age in years). MCH changes similarly. RDW remains normal.

[‡]These values are for whites only. Normal values for blacks are $5.2 \pm 2.3 \times 10^{9}/l$.

subject whose mean cell volume has always been 93 femtoliters (fl), a change to a "normal" (by reference range) 85 fl indicates a disorder. For the subject whose MCV always has been 85 fl, the same value is truly normal.

Children have MCV values less than adults'. The cause of this microcytosis does not seem to be mainly iron deficiency, but remains unclear. A method to estimate normal MCV for a given pediatric age is shown in table 2.1.

The RBC, MCV, platelet count, mean platelet volume (MPV), red cell distribution width (RDW), and WBC all are measured directly from the cell counting and sizing. The Hb is measured directly. The other values are derived from these:

hematocrit (Hct) = RBC × MCV
mean cell hemoglobin (MCH) = Hb/RBC
mean cell hemoglobin concentration (MCHC) =
  Hb/(RBC × MCV)

The histogram of red cell volume distribution is generated in several automated instruments, but is not yet always reported with the numerical results. However, a few disorders do require examination of the red cell histogram for best diagnosis of the disorder.

In practice the hemoglobin and hematocrit, although measured differently, should reflect the same biologic variable—that is, the relative concentration of red cells or hemoglobin in an aliquot of blood. Except in the rare event of a greatly abnormal MCHC, the Hb and Hct will vary similarly, so only one need be used. Hb is directly and precisely measured, and so this is probably the preferable choice.

2.2 Nondiscrete Heterogeneity

We often use the coefficient of variation (CV) to describe how reproducible repetitive measurement is. The reproducibility of values among a cell population reflects not only variability in the measurement but also biologic heterogeneity of the cells. Biologic heterogeneity can be of two kinds: discrete (having more than one subgroup), or nondiscrete (having one subgroup). Understanding the cause of changes in nondiscrete heterogeneity is crucial to understanding cell volume histograms.

All products undergo some form of "quality control": those failing pre-established criteria are kept back from distribution. The criteria cannot be too loose (the product is too variable to function acceptably) or too strict (the product is too costly to be practical). To use a marketplace analogy: stud lumber is a cheap material for building house walls. Few people would pay extra to have stud lumber finished to furniture-maker precision, because this is no benefit to the wall. Similarly, few would buy studs too irregular to frame a wall, no matter how low the price. The lumberyard offers studs just similar enough to do the job required. A similar trade-off is seen in red cells. Cells excessively heterogeneous in size would not present a reliable amount of oxygen-diffusion surface to the capillary endothelium. On the other hand, the more rigidly that red cell size is controlled, the greater the proportion that would be rejected as outside the defined limits (by the bone marrow sinusoids or the spleen) and quickly destroyed. Ineffective erythropoiesis and splenic culling are physiologic costs. The heterogeneity of a red cell property, therefore, is the result of a balance of acceptable function versus the cost of quality control.

The degree of heterogeneity of a cell property may be viewed as proportional to the importance of that variable in cell function. To return to the analogy: there is much leeway for color difference among studs, because they won't be seen under the finished wall. In contrast, there is little leeway in stud width, because that governs the surface of the wall being framed. Similarly, there is far less variation in hemoglobin concentration than in red cell size, suggesting that hemoglobin concentration has the more critical role in red cell function (Bessman, Hurley, and Groves 1983). Not surprisingly, in nucleated cells the heterogeneity of DNA content is almost nil, reflecting the central importance of DNA.

Red cell volume distribution in normals is essentially symmetrical, and can be analyzed by either a Gaussian or a log-normal model (fig. 2.1) (van Assendelft and England 1982). Most instruments use the Gaussian model. The absolute value reported for the coefficient of variation varies according to the program of the different standard instruments. Therefore, each laboratory

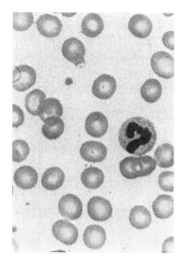

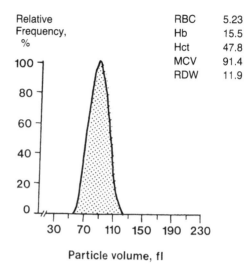

RBC	5.23
Hb	15.5
Hct	47.8
MCV	91.4
RDW	11.9

Relative Frequency, %

Particle volume, fl

FIGURE 2.1

Distribution of red cell volume in a normal subject. The automated blood count shows the RBC, MCV, Hb, and RDW (the measured variables—the others are calculated from these), the Hct, and the red cell volume distribution histogram, which is essentially symmetrical. The peripheral blood smear is for a normal subject. Variation in cell size and shape is apparent but is not abnormal. The shaded histogram likewise shows a normal degree of variation. It will be repeated in subsequent figures as a representative normal pattern against which abnormal histograms are shown. Coulter histograms have a slight right skew; Ortho, a slight left skew (see Appendix B).

should know its machine's values in normals. The values described here were determined on a Coulter Counter Model S-Plus IV, in which normal red cell volume CV is 13.2 ± 1.6 percent (Bessman, Gilmer, and Gardner 1983). In the Coulter series, CV of red cell size is reported as "red cell distribution width," or RDW. When a similar index becomes available on other instruments the name may be different, or the name may be the same but the actual measurement be different. The coefficient of variation is the ratio of standard deviation (width of the histogram) to the mean red cell volume (MCV). The index of red cell heterogeneity should not be simply the width of the histogram, because this measures only the standard deviation (SD). More useful for clinical diagnosis is the coefficient of variation. Standard deviation alone can be misleading as to whether it is normal or abnormal (table 2.2). Thus, a given SD may be normal or abnormal depending on MCV. If only the SD of red cell distribution is reported, the user must calculate CV in order to get the benefit of this measurement. Unlike most variables,

TABLE 2.2 The Difference between
Standard Deviation and Coefficient of Variation

Item	Width of Histogram		CV or RDW (%)
	MCV (mean) (fl)	(SD) (fl)	
Normal subject	81	10.1	12.5
Normal subject	99	12.4	12.5
Iron deficiency	81	12.5	15.4*
Iron deficiency	65	10.1	15.5*
Thalassemia minor	65	8.1	12.5
Folate deficiency	120	20.0	26.6*
Aplastic anemia	120	15.0	12.5

*Abnormal
Note: The text discussion is based exclusively on the coefficient of variation. A red cell called "RDW" that is based on the standard deviation will not give the distinctions shown in the text.

in which there are both abnormally high and abnormally low values, no disorder is known to have abnormally low RDW.

The peripheral blood smear in normal subjects shows a clear, but modest heterogeneity of red cell size (fig. 2.1). When quantitated, the variation of red cell area on a smear parallels that of red cell volume. Excessive heterogeneity on the blood smear is termed *anisocytosis,* the visual equivalent of increased CV. Price-Jones published an extensive experience of red blood cell size distribution based on quantitative light microscopy—measuring red cell diameters with an optical micrometer (1922). The difficulty of this manual technique hindered much further development of red cell distribution analysis until the introduction of automated instruments.

The histogram's shape varies slightly among instruments (fig. 2.1), probably due to mechanical differences (van Assendelft and England 1982; England 1984). Generally symmetrical histograms are used for illustration.

TABLE 2.3 Classification of Anemias Based on MCV and RDW

MCV Low		MCV Normal		MCV High	
RDW Normal	RDW High	RDW Normal	RDW High	RDW Normal	RDW High
Chronic disease	Iron deficiency	Normal	Early or mixed nutritional deficiency	Aplastic anemia	Folate or vitamin B_{12} deficiency
Nonanemic heterozygous thalassemia	Hb S-α or β thalassemia	Chronic disease	Anemic abnormal hemoglobin		Sickle cell anemia (⅓ of cases)
Children	Hb H	Nonanemic hemoglobin or enzyme abnormality	Myelofibrosis		Immune hemolytic anemia
		Splenectomy	Sideroblastic		Cold agglutinins
		CLL (except extreme high lymphocyte number)	Myelodysplasia		Preleukemia
		Acute blood loss			Newborn

Note: Chronic liver disease, chronic myelogenous leukemia, and cytotoxic chemotherapy may be associated with high or normal MCV, and high or normal RDW.

2.3 Initial Classification of Red Cell Disorder by Red Cell Size and Heterogeneity

Anemias have been classified by two main methods: the "morphologic" (Wintrobe 1981), in which red cell size—MCV—is the primary classifier; and the "physiologic" (Hillman and Finch 1969; Perrotta and Finch 1972), in which the amount of reticulocyte production distinguishes between hypoproliferative and hemolytic disorders. However, the reticulocyte count has a high duplicate error (Couch and Kaplow 1985). Also, because this test is not automated it costs more time and money. The classification shown below uses two automated indices: MCV and RDW. The reticulocyte count then can be used as needed to supplement this classification (Bessman 1986).

Table 2.3 illustrates the classification of anemias made possible by MCV and heterogeneity, or red cell distribution width (RDW). Six, rather than three, classifications now are possible from the initial automated blood count alone: there is a shorter list of possibilities for a given set of data, and disorders not included in previous classifications (e.g., early nutritional deficiency, red cell fragmentation) can be identified by the automated data alone. It is apparent that although the categories are based on morphologic criteria, the groupings that result are based on the physiologic distinctions that have been made in the past by reticulocyte counting.

Nutritional disorders, independent of MCV, have increased heterogeneity.

Hypoproliferative disorders, independent of MCV, have normal heterogeneity.

Hemolytic disorders, independent of MCV, have heterogeneity that is increased in direct proportion to the degree of anemia caused by the disorder.

Table 2.4 uses the same classification as table 2.3, but reorganized to emphasize physiologic distinctions.

We have found that mean cell hemoglobin concentration is abnormal in less than 1 percent of hospitalized subjects. About two-thirds of abnormal MCHC values are caused by iron deficiency, but only about 20 percent of iron deficient subjects have a low MCHC (Gottfried 1979). Therefore, low MCHC is a poor discriminant of iron deficiency. Most other causes of abnormal MCHC are artifactual, and, in practice, MCHC may be most valuable as a clue to artifact. When MCHC is normal, then MCH will parallel MCV and therefore adds little information; likewise, Hct will parallel Hb and only one value is needed. Therefore, the discussion of red cell disorders focuses primarily on the two directly measured RBC indices, MCV and RDW.

TABLE 2.4 The Morphophysiologic Classification of Red Cell Disorders

Anemia	MCV Low	MCV Normal	MCV High
Hypoproliferative disorders: RDW is always *normal*	Chronic disease	Chronic disease	Aplastic anemia
Nutritional disorders: RDW is always *high*	Iron deficiency	Early iron, folate, or vitamin B_{12} deficiency	Folate or vitamin B_{12} deficiency
	Sideroblastic	Sideroblastic	Sideroblastic
Hemolytic disorders: RDW is *increased proportionally* to the degree of *anemia*			
RDW normal:	Thalassemia trait or carrier	AS, AC, other hemoglobinopathies without anemia	
		Enzyme or membrane defects without chronic anemia	
RDW high:	Thalassemia intermedia or H disease	Hb SS	Hb SS
	S-β thalassemia		Immune hemolytic anemia
	SS and α-thalassemia		
Artifacts that have a high RDW and an abnormal histogram	Red cell fragments	Red cell fragments Posttransfusion	Cold agglutinins CLL Hyperglycemia

Source: Adapted from Bessman, Gilmer, and Gardner 1983.

2.4 Microcytic Disorders

2.4.1 *Normal Heterogeneity: Thalassemia*

The recent advances that have been made in the molecular genetics of thalassemia are well detailed elsewhere (Bunn and Forget 1985). In brief, the thalassemias are imbalances between production of the α and the non-α (β, γ, and δ)

TABLE 2.5 Red Cell Indices in the Heterozygous Thalassemias

Alleles	Name	Hb (g/dl)	RBC ($10^{12}/l$)	MCV (fl)	CV or RDW (%)
αα/αα or ββ	Normal	16.1±2.0	5.41±0.72	90±10	13.3±1.5
αα/α− or β+	α Silent carrier/ heterozygous β+	15.5±2.0	5.52±0.76	81±10	13.5±1.5
αα/− − or β−	Trait (α or β)	14.5±2.0	5.96±0.81	72±10	14.1±1.5
α−/− − or + −	H disease/β-Thalassemia intermedia	9.0±3.0	4.56±0.61	63±10	16.7±1.8
− −/− − or − −	Hydrops or β-Thalasse-mia major	Rarely seen untransfused			

Note: − indicates a deleted or nonfunctional locus; +, a hypofunctional locus; hemoglobin and RBC count are for males. (Based on our data and Steinberg et al. 1984.)

globin chains: the imbalance is caused by deletion or abnormality of one or more of the four α or two β alleles. The alteration in the blood counts is summarized by table 2.5.

Table 2.5 illustrates that the phenotypic abnormality (microcytosis) is overlaid on the substantial variation of MCV that is found among normal subjects. Each single α-locus deletion on average reduces mean cell volume approximately 9 fl. The mean normal value for MCV is 90 fl. Therefore, in more than half of subjects the 9 fl reduction of a single α-locus deletion will not bring MCV below 80 fl, the bottom of the "normal" range. These subjects are truly "silent carriers." Furthermore, in a few cases, even the average 18 fl reduction of MCV caused by two α-locus deletions ("trait") does not bring MCV below normal. A similar situation is seen in heterozygous β-thalassemia, in which one β-locus deletion causes a phenotypic change similar to two α-locus deletions.

The RDW of the red cells is generally normal in the lesser degrees of thalassemia accompanied by low MCV but not anemia (fig. 2.2)

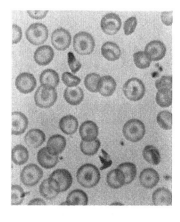

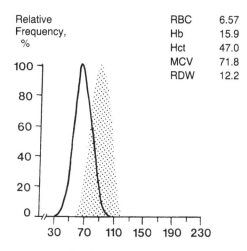

RBC	6.57
Hb	15.9
Hct	47.0
MCV	71.8
RDW	12.2

Particle volume, fl

FIGURE 2.2

Heterozygous α-thalassemia (two-locus deletion). MCV is reduced, red cell count is increased, and RDW is normal. The blood smear may or may not show target cells or basophilic stippling. Heterogeneity of red cell size is not increased in these subjects with normal levels of hemoglobin.

(Bessman and Feinstein 1979; Johnson, Tegos, and Beutler 1983). Only to the extent that the heterozygous thalassemia (rather than concurrent chronic disease) causes a modest anemia will RDW rise slightly (Kaye and Alter 1985). Although the peripheral blood may show apparent slight variation of size in red cells of silent carrier or trait patients, usually this reflects increased variation of shape (targeting, primarily) rather than of either size or hemoglobin content.

The diagnosis of heterozygous thalassemia (silent carrier or trait) can therefore be made presumptively in the nonanemic subject by low MCV and normal RDW. Confirmatory tests are hemoglobin electrophoresis with hemoglobin A_2 quantitation for β-thalassemias (about $50 and two days) and DNA analysis for α-thalassemia (available only at a few centers). Iron deficiency may be excluded by iron-binding studies or ferritin (each, requiring about $50 and one to two days). If concurrent iron deficiency is present, RDW is increased because of the iron deficiency; hemoglobin A_2 percentage also may no longer be increased in subjects with hetero-

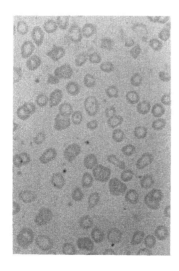

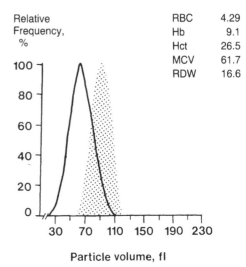

RBC	4.29
Hb	9.1
Hct	26.5
MCV	61.7
RDW	16.6

Particle volume, fl

FIGURE 2.3
*Hemoglobin H disease.
There is anemia, marked
microcytosis, and an in-
creased RDW. As dis-
cussed in the text, a
hemoglobinopathy asso-
ciated with anemia can
be expected to have an
increased RDW.*

zygous β-thalassemia. An important benefit of
identifying heterozygous thalassemia is to pre-
vent the needless investigation, worry, and ex-
pense caused by confusion with the microcytosis
of iron deficiency, and to improve genetic coun-
seling. Note that there is no way to detect from
the blood count or smear those subjects with
heterozygous thalassemia and a normal MCV.

In contrast, patients with hemoglobin H disease or β-thalassemia intermedia have frank
anemia, and as in other hemoglobinopathies,
increased RDW accompanies disorders severe
enough to create anemia (fig. 2.3). The peripheral blood smear shows marked microcytosis
with pronounced heterogeneity of size (Bessman
and Feinstein 1979).

2.4.2 *Increased Heterogeneity: Iron Deficiency*

Iron deficiency is the cause of the great majority
of cases of low MCV; essentially the balance of
cases are heterozygous thalassemia, discussed
in the previous section (Fairbanks and Beutler
1983). Iron deficiency already is well established
by the time the MCV falls, because first the bone

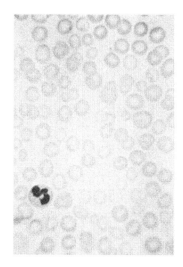

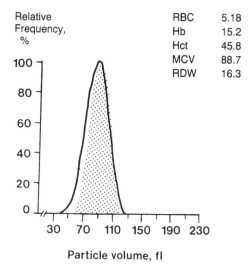

RBC	5.18
Hb	15.2
Hct	45.8
MCV	88.7
RDW	16.3

FIGURE 2.4

Early iron deficiency. Mean size still is in the normal range and anemia is not yet apparent. Even so, RDW already is increased: the histogram is unimodal but is wider than normal. The peripheral smear shows only increased red cell heterogeneity.

marrow is depleted of iron stores, and only then is erythropoiesis altered. As iron deficiency persists, progressively smaller cells are made. The normal red cell's life span is about 120 days; therefore, even when abnormally small red cells first are being produced, for the next month or so the remaining normal size cells are in the majority so MCV changes little (fig. 2.4). The more severe and longstanding the iron deficiency, the smaller the MCV tends to be (fig. 2.5). Iron deficiency usually is progressive or fluctuating in severity. The peripheral blood includes red cells that reflect 120 days of this changing erythropoiesis: either progressively smaller cells or cells of fluctuating size. Therefore, increased heterogeneity of size is seen on the peripheral blood smear (anisocytosis) and on the volume distribution histogram (increased RDW). There is increased RDW even in subjects with early iron deficiency, in which hemoglobin and MCV still are within the normal range (e.g., early in gastrointestinal bleeding, or during the course of phlebotomy for polycythemia) (Bessman 1980a; England and Down 1974). Increased RDW that

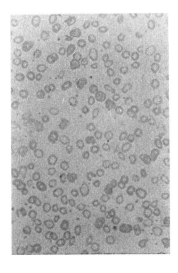

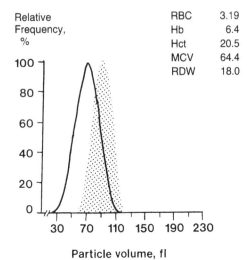

Relative Frequency, %

RBC	3.19
Hb	6.4
Hct	20.5
MCV	64.4
RDW	18.0

Particle volume, fl

FIGURE 2.5
Advanced iron deficiency. This is what is usually shown as an example of this disease. Anemia is present, MCV is very low, and the smear is very abnormal. Again the RDW is abnormally high; the histogram remains abnormal. The diagnosis is easily made at this point, but earlier identification (e.g., fig. 2.4) would improve management.

accompanies otherwise normal red cell values distinguishes early iron deficiency from normal (McClure, Custer, and Bessman 1985). Increased RDW combined with low MCV distinguishes iron deficiency from nonanemic heterozygous thalassemia, in which the RDW is normal (Bessman 1980a; Bessman and Feinstein 1979). Calculations based on the MCV and red cell count and/or hemoglobin have been proposed to distinguish between thalassemia and iron deficiency (England and Fraser 1979). These assume that in thalassemia the red cell count is normal to high, and in iron deficiency the red cell count is low. These indices can distinguish heterozygous thalassemia only from obvious advanced iron deficiency, and are less reliable than the RDW in distinguishing the two diseases when the red cell count is low-normal to normal (Bessman and Feinstein 1979).

Iron stores may be depleted before erythropoiesis becomes abnormal at all. Depleted iron stores alone will not produce abnormal RDW, MCV, or Hb (see table 2.6 on p. 28).

Recovery from iron deficiency begins with re-

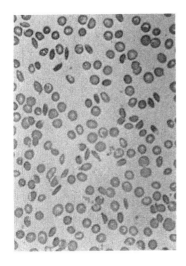

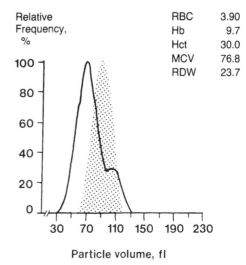

Relative Frequency, %		RBC	3.90
		Hb	9.7
		Hct	30.0
		MCV	76.8
		RDW	23.7

Particle volume, fl

FIGURE 2.6

Recovery from iron deficiency. This is the blood picture ten days after that in figure 2.5. The red cell count is increasing, MCV is not yet normal, and two populations of red cells are seen—preexisting microcytes, and newly-formed normocytes. The two populations are distinguished easily on the red cell histogram but not so easily on the peripheral blood smear. Contrast this pattern with figure 2.7.

ticulocytosis three to five days after iron replenishment is started. If the MCV is low to begin with, a distinctly different-size population of cells will appear concurrent with the appearance of reticulocytes. The second population will be normal in size if the iron deficiency was the only problem. However, MCV will remain low for several weeks until the newly formed red cells outnumber sufficiently the remaining microcytes (fig. 2.6). In contrast, a concomitant macrocytic disorder is found in 10–20 percent of patients with iron deficiency. In these patients, the new cells will reflect the unsuspected macrocytic disorder and MCV will progressively rise through the normal range to an abnormal high value (fig. 2.7) (Bessman 1977a). In many instances of mixed iron and folate deficiency, the macrocytic and microcytic disorders cancel each other out enough to cause a normal MCV (see section 2.5.2.2) (Spivak 1982).

Aluminum excess may interfere with iron metabolism and produce any degree of anemia and microcytosis (O'Hare and Murnaghan 1982). The mechanism may be direct competition with iron

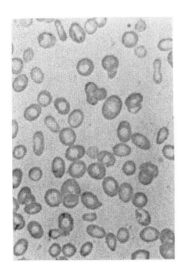

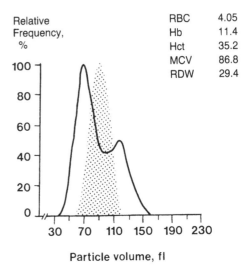

RBC	4.05	
Hb	11.4	
Hct	35.2	
MCV	86.8	
RDW	29.4	

Relative Frequency, %

Particle volume, fl

FIGURE 2.7

*Recovery from iron defi-
ciency, ten days after
treatment was begun. In
contrast to figure 2.6, in
this case the new cells
are macrocytic: note the
right peak has a mean
value of 117 fl. This
macrocytic response indi-
cates an unmasked
underlying macrocytic
disorder. Use of the his-
togram allows this analy-
sis even though the MCV
is only 86.8 fl. Again the
two populations cannot
be well distinguished from
the blood smear.*

for transferrin (Trapp 1983). The RDW is increased.

Chronic infection may cause malutilization of
iron as well as erythroid suppression. In patients
with anemia due to chronic infection, increased
RDW may be caused by iron malutilization, but
other causes, such as liver disease, also should
be sought (Baynes et al. 1986).

Mean cell hemoglobin concentration and mean
cell hemoglobin also often fall in iron deficiency.
In marked iron deficiency, the red cell shape and
deformability are abnormal. For example, if the
"true" mean cell size in a severe case of iron
deficiency is 70 fl, but abnormal shape and deformability cause an artifactual 5 percent increase in nominal volume (Bator et al. 1984), the
reported MCV will be 73.5 fl. Because MCH is
unaffected by this artifact, MCH/MCV will be
reduced by 5 percent and MCHC will be artifactually 5 percent low (e.g., 31.5 percent instead of 33 percent). Even so, MCHC is normal
often enough in iron deficiency that some laboratories recommend not using MCHC in routine
diagnosis (Gottfried 1979). This level of interaction of shape and size has been best charac-

terized in Coulter instruments, but probably is similar in other instruments. It is far less than the degree to which abnormal red cell packing caused artifactual MCHC in manual methods. Only extremely abnormal red cells, such as in homozygous S disease, may have a substantial shape-deformability artifact. In these cases, other blood count abnormalities are likely to be diagnostic.

2.5 Normocytic Disorders

2.5.1 *Normal Heterogeneity*

2.5.1.1 Chronic Disease

The anemia associated with certain diseases is generally hypoproliferative: a relative failure of erythroid stem cells to proliferate rather than a specific deficiency of some cytoplasmic or nuclear component. The proliferative deficiency may result from impaired erythropoietin production (renal disease) or from less well characterized causes (e.g., hypothyroidism, chronic infection). Likewise, many drugs suppress erythropoiesis, either as a recognized though unwanted side effect (e.g., chloramphenicol) or a part of planned marrow toxicity (e.g., anti-leukemic chemotherapy). Because the deficiency is in the proliferation rather than the maturation of the cell, the abnormality is essentially of cell number. Cell size is little changed, and cellular heterogeneity is not increased in such situations. The peripheral blood smear reflects the normal cell size and heterogeneity (fig. 2.8).

Anemia of chronic disease generally is associated with normal MCV, but there are many series that report microcytosis also. In our series, subjects with anemia (<10g/dl) caused by chronic renal failure had MCV values of 85.8 ± 11.3 fl. Most were normocytic, but the mean value was lower; about 15 percent had an MCV below 80 fl. There was no difference in volume heterogeneity between the patients at the top

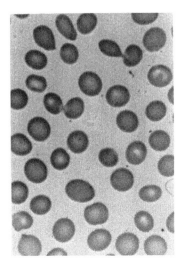

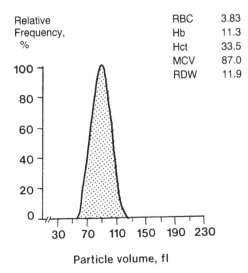

Relative Frequency, %

RBC	3.83
Hb	11.3
Hct	33.5
MCV	87.0
RDW	11.9

Particle volume, fl

FIGURE 2.8
Chronic disease. All values are normal except for anemia. The peripheral blood smear and histogram resemble those seen in normal subjects.

and the bottom of the MCV range. Thus, in patients with low MCV, increased RDW distinguishes iron deficiency from either heterozygous thalassemia or chronic disease. In patients with normal MCV, increased RDW distinguishes iron deficiency from chronic disease (Bessman, Gilmer, and Gardner 1983; Kaye and Alter 1985).

Chronic liver disease or chronic alcohol abuse is slightly different in that the MCV is normal to high. In 36 patients in whom folate deficiency or hemolytic disease was excluded, the MCV was 93.3 ± 11.6 fl. In the minority of cases in which macrocytosis occurred, it may have been due to changes in the red cell membrane (Bator et al. 1984) that alter the red cell deformability to produce a slightly increased apparent MCV. However, in chronic liver disease, various combinations of slight hemolysis; red cell membrane changes; folate deficiency; and altered deformability may make the cause of slight macrocytosis difficult to pinpoint (Chalmers et al. 1979). Likewise, whereas most such subjects have normal RDW, about 30 percent have an increased RDW (Bessman, Gilmer, and Gardner 1983). Because of the multifactorial nature of chronic liver disease, MCV alone is not a good classifier. Therefore, adding RDW does not bring these patients into a single classification (McDonald et al. 1984). Note that these changes may occur even without anemia.

Thyroid disease is remarkable in that hypothyroidism is associated with a modest increase in MCV, and hyperthyroidism, with a slight decrease. Often the change will be within the normal range, but abnormal for the individual; less often, there will be overt macro- or microcytosis. The RDW remains normal. The MCV returns to normal after successful therapy of the thyroid disorder. The size disorder therefore seems related to the thyroid's metabolism, perhaps via alteration of red cell membrane lipids (Davidson et al. 1984).

2.5.1.2 Acute Blood Loss

Unless there is transfusion of red cells, acute blood loss does not immediately alter MCV or RDW, since the remaining cells are unchanged. Of course, if previous blood loss already had made the patient iron deficient at the time of acute blood loss, the MCV and RDW would reflect this. About four days after the acute blood loss, increased reticulocytosis will begin. Reticulocytes are on average about 8 percent larger than the cells into which they mature (Clarkson and Moore 1976; Gilmer and Koepke 1976) (fig. 2.9). Therefore, even a substantial increase in reticulocytes will not change the MCV or RDW. A simple calculation emphasizes this point: If the mature red cells have a volume of 90 fl, and the reticulocytes are 8 percent larger, then a 20 percent reticulocytosis will raise the whole-blood MCV to only 91.6 fl. Conversely, if an increase of 10 fl in the MCV is to be attributed to marked reticulocytosis (e.g., 20 percent), then:

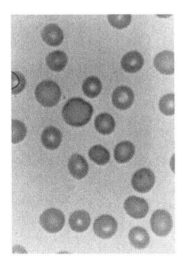

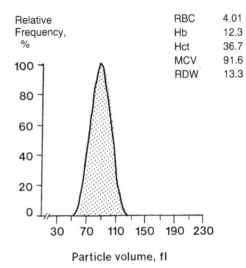

	RBC	4.01
	Hb	12.3
	Hct	36.7
	MCV	91.6
	RDW	13.3

Particle volume, fl

FIGURE 2.9

Acute blood loss, four days before these data. On this day the reticulocytes are 10 percent of the red cells. Reticulocytes are apparent on the peripheral blood smear: they are 8 percent larger than mature cells and also are flatter. However, no second population is seen on the histogram, and the MCV and RDW both are normal.

(80 percent mature cells at 90 fl)
+ (20 percent reticulocytes at volume X)
must equal
(100 percent total cells at 100 fl)

Solving for this equation yields a reticulocyte mean volume of 140 fl. Figure 2.9 shows how unlikely this is.

Hemoglobin Pasadena is an unstable hemolytic anemia with normal hemoglobin amount, MCV, and RDW but 15 percent reticulocytes. These reticulocytes, not apparently different in size from mature cells, do not cause macrocytosis (Johnson et al. 1980). When high MCV is accompanied by increased reticulocytes, the mature red cells also will be macrocytic (see section 2.6.1.2). Therefore, reticulocytes per se do not substantially change either the MCV or the RDW. An increase in MCV due to reticulocytosis often is described (Williams et al. 1983; Wintrobe 1981). Generally this is seen only when there is prolonged "stress" erythropoiesis (erythroblast maturation is altered to speed red cell production). In humans, such "stress" erythropoiesis

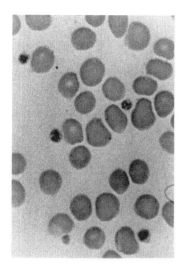

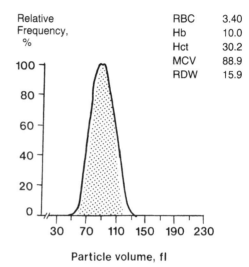

RBC	3.40
Hb	10.0
Hct	30.2
MCV	88.9
RDW	15.9

Particle volume, fl

FIGURE 2.10

Transfusion. The values for the patient's cells were: MCV 86.3 fl, RDW 12.8 percent. The values of the transfused cells were: MCV 94.7 fl, RDW 13.3 percent. The two populations cannot be distinguished on either the blood smear or the histogram, but the overlap produces an increased RDW. In many cases the difference between donor and recipient MCV is so small that the RDW is normal.

is found almost exclusively in immune hemolytic anemia (see section 2.6.1.2). If there is not immune hemolytic anemia, a high MCV is very unlikely to be explained by reticulocytosis; other causes should be sought (van Assendelft and England 1982).

Transfusion will affect both MCV and RDW to the extent that the transfused blood differs in MCV from that of the recipient. Because blood banks depend increasingly on volunteer donors, MCV tends to be normal (80–99 fl in 143 of 143 units tested in our blood bank). However, even within this normal range, a difference of 10 fl between donor and recipient may be present. This degree of difference will cause an increased RDW (fig. 2.10), but the two populations will overlap enough that the histogram will not have two peaks. However, if the donor and recipient red cells are more similar in size, the RDW will remain normal.

2.5.1.3 Nonimmune Hemolysis

Patients with increased reticulocytosis and normal to slightly reduced hemoglobin levels due to

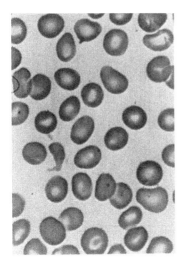

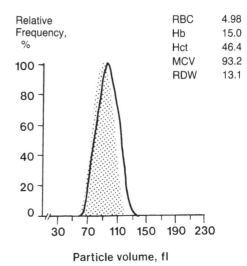

RBC	4.98
Hb	15.0
Hct	46.4
MCV	93.2
RDW	13.1

Particle volume, fl

FIGURE 2.11
Glucose-6-phosphate de-hydrogenase deficiency. Hemoglobin, MCV, and RDW all are normal, despite the patient's chronic hemolysis with a reticulocytosis of 3–6 percent.

glucose-6-phosphate dehydrogenase, pyruvate kinase deficiency (in our experience, n=6), or hereditary spherocytosis (n=5) have a normal RDW. Generally, they also have a normal MCV. Since the increase in compensatory erythropoiesis is less than in severe immune hemolysis, the reticulocytosis is not of the "stress" variety (see above). However, polychromatophilic reticulocytes may be prominent on the peripheral blood smear (fig. 2.11). Even during a hemolytic crisis, so long as it is short-lived, MCV does not rise. Only when the red cell destruction lasts for weeks does the pattern of erythropoiesis change to the "stress" macrocytes. Patients with hereditary spherocytosis usually have MCV in the low normal range: 83.6 ± 11.4 fl. In our series of five patients, MCHC is often but not always elevated. While these slight abnormalities may be due to loss of cell volume by splenic remodeling, red cell shape also may play a part. The "shape factor" used to translate machine measurements into the cell volume that is reported assumes a nonspherical erythrocyte that is incompletely sphered by the diluent. Because of this assumption, the spherocyte's more complete sphering and altered deformability causes artifactually a slightly low volume measurement. Because MCH is accurate, MCHC will be falsely increased to the extent that the MCV is falsely low.

2.5.1.4 Splenectomy

Splenectomy done for splenic trauma or incidental to surgery yields (in 14 subjects of our experience) normal MCV and RDW unchanged from the presurgery value. Thus, the presence of Howell-Jolly bodies does not apparently affect these indices. However, if the splenectomy is done to alleviate a hemolytic disorder such as hereditary spherocytosis, the MCV will not change but RDW may increase slightly. If the splenectomy is done in the presence of a hematologic malignancy, especially in subjects receiving cytotoxic chemotherapy (e.g., chronic myelogenous leukemia, hairy cell leukemia, lymphoma), the RDW may be markedly increased despite a normal MCV and hemoglobin. In such patients the preoperative RDW also is increased, though less markedly so. Splenectomy allows the survival in the peripheral blood of cells with abnormal properties. The change in RDW after splenectomy suggests the degree to which abnormal erythrocytes, previously culled by the spleen, no longer are after splenectomy.

2.5.2 *Increased Heterogeneity*

2.5.2.1 Early Nutritional Deficiency

As noted in section 2.4.2, even when iron deficiency is so early that MCV and Hb still are normal, the RDW usually is increased. In an inpatient population of subjects with otherwise normal automated blood counts, an isolated high RDW indicates iron deficiency perhaps two-thirds of the time (McClure, Custer, and Bessman 1985). Occasionally, because the range of normal values is broad enough, a subject with base-

TABLE 2.6 Progressive Stages of Iron Deficiency

Stage	Iron Stores*	RDW	MCV	Hb
Depletion	Reduced	Normal	Normal	Normal
Heterogeneous	Reduced	High	Normal	Normal
Microcytic	Reduced	High	Low	Normal
Anemic	Reduced	High	Low	Low

*Marrow stainable iron; ferritin; or transferrin saturation.

line low-normal Hb or MCV, and low-normal RDW values will have Hb or MCV fall below the normal range before RDW rises above the normal range. Our and others' unpublished experience suggests this occurs in <5 percent of cases. Also, marrow and serum iron depletion develop before any abnormal erythropoiesis appears (Fairbanks and Beutler 1983). Therefore, all cases of early iron depletion will not be detected by increased RDW. However, increased RDW will reveal far more and earlier cases of iron deficiency than abnormal MCV, Hb, or MCHC. In an ambulatory population, approximately 15 percent of women 18–50 years old will have iron deficiency detectable by increased RDW; less than 5 percent will have iron deficiency detectable by low MCV or Hb (unpublished data). The usual progression of iron deficiency can be characterized as shown in table 2.6.

2.5.2.2 Sickle Cell Anemia and Other Hemoglobinopathies

Among the hemoglobinopathies there is an inverse correlation between hemoglobin level (or packed cell volume) and RDW (fig. 2.12) (Bessman 1980a). The cause of this relation is not known. Unlike the progressive nature of the nutritional deficiencies described above, hemoglobinopathies generally are constant throughout life (β-chain variants become phenotypically constant only during infancy, after the hemo-

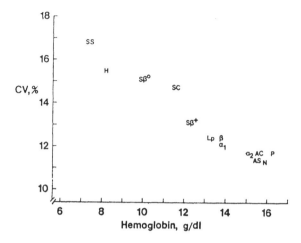

FIGURE 2.12
*The relation between ane-
mia and red cell volume
CV (RDW) in hemo-
globinopathies. If the
bone marrow can com-
pensate for the hemo-
globinopathy enough to
allow a normal hemo-
globin (on average, 16
g/dl in men), CV is nor-
mal. The abbreviations
represent subjects with
hemoglobins SS, SC, AS,
AC, and Pasadena (P);
with heterozygous β, α_2,
α_1, H, and Lepore (Lp)
thalassemias; hemoglobin
$S\beta^0$ or $S\beta^+$-thalassemia;
and normal (N) subjects.
Source: Bessman 1980a.*

globin F abates). One possible explanation is
that heterogeneity of red cell production does not
change in hemoglobinopathies, but quality control of the red cells progressively is sacrificed as
anemia worsens. The physical site of quality
control is at least in part in the bone marrow
sinusoids and spleen, both of which can cull
cells that fail to meet criteria for passage. Criteria may include, but may not be limited to:
cell size, deformability, and metabolic reserve.
However, it is unknown whether the criteria for
passage through spleen or sinusoid can be
changed by anemia.

A second possible explanation for the relation
between anemia and anisocytosis is that red cell
heterogeneity *is* inherently increased proportional
to the degree of abnormality of hemoglobin synthesis, and that quality control is constant. With
an increased heterogeneity of red cell production, a constant quality control would cull a
progressively greater proportion of cells either in
the bone marrow or spleen, and a smaller frac-
tion of red cells would circulate. A marked increase in RDW can occur in the presence of
either splenomegaly (hemoglobin H disease) or
functional asplenia (adult SS disease). These

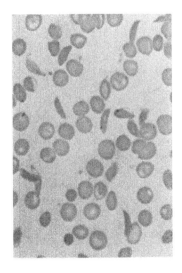

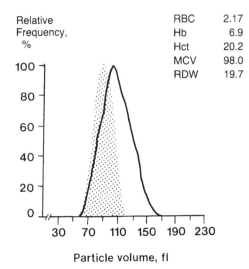

Relative Frequency, %

Particle volume, fl

RBC	2.17
Hb	6.9
Hct	20.2
MCV	98.0
RDW	19.7

FIGURE 2.13
Sickle cell anemia. The red cell count is markedly reduced. MCV is high-normal and RDW is high. The blood smear shows typical features: poly-chromasia and many sickled cells.

two explanations for the relation of anemia and RDW are at this point only speculative. An element of both mechanisms may be present. As noted earlier, reticulocytosis per se does not cause increased MCV or RDW, as illustrated by hemoglobin Pasadena (Johnson et al. 1980). Also, among the anemic hemoglobinopathies, RDW is increased whether MCV is low (H disease) or high (SS disease).

In sickle cell anemia, anisocytosis is obvious in the peripheral blood smear as well as the automated blood count (fig. 2.13). The MCV is 98 ± 15 fl, and nearly half such patients will have an abnormally high MCV (Serjeant et al. 1981). However, this should be viewed as a continuum: in our study of 152 patients with hemoglobin SS, there was no correlation between MCV and other variables such as hemoglobin level, reticulocyte count, hemoglobin (Hb) F level, or RDW. A recent study (Steinberg et al. 1984) suggests there is a higher MCV in patients with increased Hb F. The macrocytosis may be in part a "stress" reticulocytosis (Finch 1982). Also, red cell deformability probably affects the

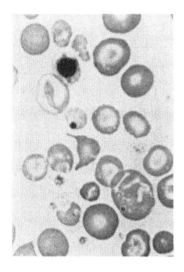

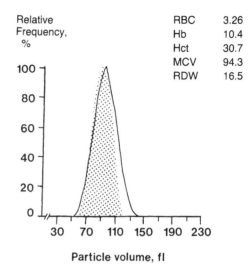

	RBC	3.26
	Hb	10.4
	Hct	30.7
	MCV	94.3
	RDW	16.5

Relative Frequency, %

Particle volume, fl

FIGURE 2.14
Hemoglobin SC disease. The red cell count is moderately reduced, the MCV is normal, and the RDW is moderately increased, consonant with the moderate degree of anemia. The blood smear shows a wide variation of cell shape peculiar to hemoglobin SC disease. The disparity in heterogeneity between blood smear and RDW is due to shape heterogeneity, which is not measured by the automated counter.

reported MCV. The reduced deformability and irregular shape (resisting sphering in the diluent that is used in the counter) of sickled cells yields a slightly high impedance value. When the "shape factor" calculation is altered to reflect the sickled cells' shape, perhaps half of the apparent macrocytosis disappears (Bator et al. 1984). Because MCH is reported correctly, the artifactually high MCV yields an artifactually low MCHC. Even so, MCHC often is increased in patients with SS (Embury et al. 1982). The RDW is consistently well above normal, and does not substantially change during sickling crises (unpublished data; S. Charache, personal communication).

Patients with SS disease and concomitant heterozygous α-thalassemia have reduced MCV (Embury et al. 1982; Higgs et al. 1982). The hemoglobin level of these patients is modestly increased, and to that extent the RDW is less increased than in other SS patients (unpublished data). Low MCV and high RDW in sickle cell anemia also can be seen when there is complicating iron deficiency: red cell indices will

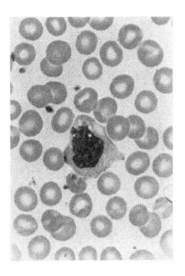

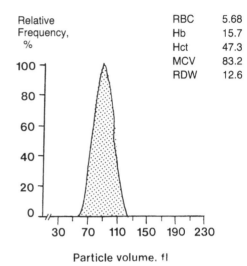

RBC	5.68
Hb	15.7
Hct	47.3
MCV	83.2
RDW	12.6

Particle volume. fl

FIGURE 2.15
Hemoglobin AS (S trait). There is no abnormality of the blood smear, blood count, or histogram. If there is an abnormality in a patient with hemoglobin AS or AC, a different cause should be sought.

not reliably distinguish these two conditions (Natta et al. 1982).

Patients who are double heterozygotes of hemoglobin SC or S-β thalassemia have peripheral blood smears that are particularly striking for apparent anisocytosis and poikilocytosis (fig. 2.14). The targeting and intracellular crystals make it easy to confuse heterogeneity of shape for heterogeneity of size. The RDW is only moderately increased and correlates with the moderate anemia most such patients have (fig. 2.12) (Bessman 1980a).

Nonanemic hemoglobinopathies are not associated with an increased RDW, whether MCV is normal (heterozygous AS or AC) or low (double heterozygotes for hemoglobin S or C and for α- or thalassemia) (fig. 2.15). If RDW is increased in a subject with hemoglobin AS or AC, then nutritional deficiency, rather than the heterozygous hemoglobinopathy, should be suspected as the cause (Hammersley et al. 1981).

The same relationship between anemia and anisocytosis is seen in hemoglobinopathies and in thalassemias. Increasing sophistication of

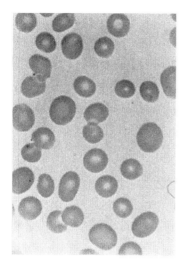

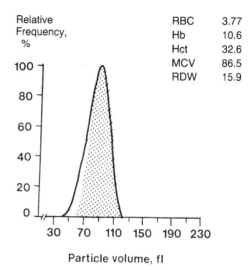

	RBC	3.77
	Hb	10.6
	Hct	32.6
	MCV	86.5
	RDW	15.9

Relative Frequency, %

Particle volume, fl

FIGURE 2.16
Mixed deficiency of folic acid and iron. The red cell count is moderately reduced, MCV is normal, and RDW moderately increased. The peripheral blood smear is abnormal only in the heterogeneity of cell size: neither megaloblastic nor iron-deficient abnormalities are apparent. The increased RDW is the only clue to abnormality.

molecular analysis suggests these two disease types are overlapping in their pathology (Steinberg and Adams 1983). Both involve abnormal globin production that is constant throughout life, accompanied by a degree of intra- and extra-medullary red cell hyperdestruction that tends to parallel the degree of anemia.

2.5.2.3 Mixed Nutritional Deficiency

Isolated iron deficiency often but not always is associated with low MCV. Isolated folate or vitamin B_{12} deficiency often is associated with high MCV. If iron deficiency and folate or vitamin B_{12} deficiency coexist, one may predominate enough to cause abnormal MCV. Otherwise, the deficiencies may together cause a normal MCV (Spivak 1982). The RDW is increased—the clue to the possibility of nutritional deficiency rather than chronic disease. Figure 2.7 shows that if one nutritional deficiency is unmasked by therapy for another that is initially more obvious, two red cell populations will appear. In contrast, if both untreated deficiencies are about equally severe there will be only a single population of cells, widely distributed (fig. 2.16). Similar values are caused by the combination of α-thalassemia and vitamin B_{12} deficiency (Green et al. 1982). The MCV may be normal, but the RDW will be increased by the vitamin B_{12} deficiency. When there is a concomitant high-RDW disorder, the normal RDW associated with heterozygous thalassemia will be obscured.

2.5.2.4 Cytotoxic Chemotherapy

Subjects receiving cytotoxic chemotherapy for malignancy or immune disorders will have either a normal or high MCV, and either a normal or high RDW. The same subjects before chemo-therapy have a normal MCV and RDW (if there is no other hematologic disorder). The degree to which MCV and/or RDW become abnormal may reflect the degree to which red cell production is affected in quality as well as in numbers by the cytotoxic agents. Many cytotoxic drugs, singly or in combination, both suppress cell production and (similar to megaloblastic nutritional deficiency) interfere with DNA synthesis. The changes in Hb, MCV, and RDW will reflect the relative degree of megaloblastic and hypoproliferative changes. Therefore, no single combination of MCV and RDW is characteristic of chemo-therapy (McDonald et al. 1984; Bessman 1985).

2.5.2.5 Myelofibrosis and Myelodysplasia

The spleen (unless removed) generally becomes a site of extramedullary hematopoiesis in myelo-fibrosis. As this occurs, the spleen's filtering function progressively is lost, allowing immature granulocytes, nucleated red cells, and increased numbers of reticulocytes to appear in the periph-eral blood. The loss of filtration also may be a reason that the red cell volume is charac-teristically abnormally heterogeneous, yielding a high RDW (fig. 2.17). It is unknown whether splenic erythropoiesis per se differs from that in the bone marrow. Despite the nucleated red

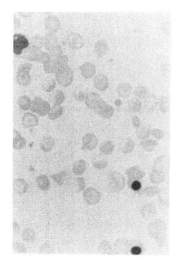

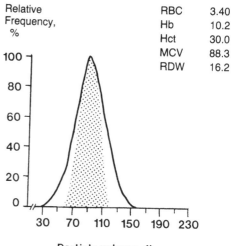

RBC	3.40
Hb	10.2
Hct	30.0
MCV	88.3
RDW	16.2

Particle volume, fl

FIGURE 2.17
Myelofibrosis. The red cell count is reduced, MCV is normal, and the RDW is increased. These data alert the clinician to the abnormality; the specific disease can be inferred from the specific changes on the blood smear: nucleated red cells, and teardrop cells.

cells and increased reticulocytes, MCV generally is normal (91 ± 13 fl in our series). In one patient with congenital myelosclerosis, androgen therapy reversed the anemia but not the red cell heterogeneity, suggesting an inherent qualitative defect of erythropoiesis that was independent of the quantitative defect.

Myelodysplastic syndromes are a diverse group of disorders. The MCV, RDW, and Hb range from near normal to markedly abnormal (McDonald et al. 1984). Preleukemia typically has a high MCV, but there is no typical pattern of cell count.

2.5.2.6 Sideroblastic Anemia

The classical description of the red cells in idiopathic sideroblastic anemia is that of a "dimorphic population" (Wintrobe 1981): both macrocytes and microcytes. The MCV has been described as low, normal, or above normal. The volume distribution histogram is always markedly widened beyond normal. Generally, there is a single peak (fig. 2.18) but occasionally there is the suggestion of two populations. Note that in

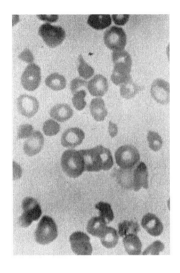

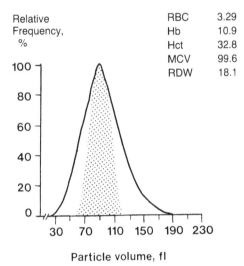

RBC	3.29
Hb	10.9
Hct	32.8
MCV	99.6
RDW	18.1

Relative Frequency, %

Particle volume, fl

FIGURE 2.18
Sideroblastic anemia. The red cell count is reduced, and RDW is increased. MCV in sideroblastic anemia is most often normal, but may be either high or low. The blood smear shows a marked variation in red cell size but the histogram rarely shows two discrete red cell populations.

the corresponding blood smear the great variation in size allows the viewer to identify both macrocytes and microcytes. However, these may be the extremes of a single widely distributed population rather than truly discrete subpopulations. In our series, MCV has ranged from 83 to 108 fl with a mean of 94 fl (Bessman, Gilmer, and Gardner 1983). In only a minority are two distinct subpopulations seen in the red cell histogram.

Ethanol-induced sideroblastic anemia has a similar picture, though this is often complicated by folate deficiency, changes of liver disease, or low-grade hemolytic anemia.

2.6 Macrocytic Disorders

2.6.1 *Normal Heterogeneity: Aplastic Anemia*

Two types of aplasia should be distinguished: (1) temporary myelosuppression from a known drug or toxin that remits when the agent is stopped; and (2) permanent aplasia determined either by idiopathic causes or by a known agent. The complete list of known drugs is well reviewed

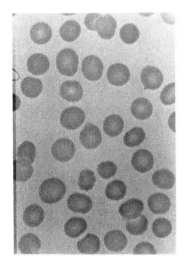

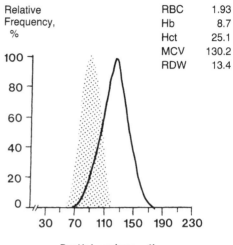

Relative Frequency, %

RBC	1.93
Hb	8.7
Hct	25.1
MCV	130.2
RDW	13.4

Particle volume, fl

FIGURE 2.19
Untransfused aplastic anemia. The hemoglobin is reduced, the MCV is increased, and RDW is normal. Aplastic anemia is typically a macrocytic, homogeneous anemia if there has been no recent transfusion.

elsewhere (Wintrobe 1981; Williams et al. 1983); chloramphenicol can cause both types.

The temporary type of aplasia may cause a profound anemia but the anemia is normocytic and has a normal RDW. This suggests that the stem cell itself is not altered qualitatively, but quantitatively. In contrast is chronic adult aplastic anemia. These patients' red cells nearly always are macrocytic, suggesting a qualitative change in the stem cell (Bessman and Gardner 1985). Reports vary as to what MCV is associated with aplastic anemia (Champlin, Ho, and Gale 1983; Rappeport and Nathan 1982; Camitta, Storb, and Thomas 1982). Patients so studied have received a variable number of red transfusions before the MCV is measured. Because transfused cells are almost always normocytic, transfusion will partially or (if >10 units in three months) may totally obscure the MCV of the patient's cells. In our patients with aplastic anemia of at least three months duration, 33 of 35 patients had an MCV >100 fl in their own cells, which could be distinguished from transfused cells by the red cell histogram. The marrow nu-

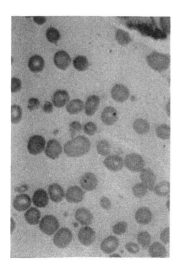

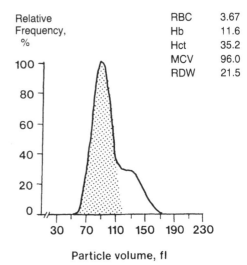

Relative Frequency, %

		RBC	3.67
		Hb	11.6
		Hct	35.2
		MCV	96.0
		RDW	21.5

Particle volume, fl

FIGURE 2.20

Transfused aplastic anemia. The MCV now is normal, in contrast to figure 2.19. Two populations of red cells are seen on the histogram: transfused normocytes and the patient's macrocytes. The reader should consider whether these two populations, so clearly distinct on the histogram, could be distinguished on the blood smear without prior knowledge of the clinical data.

cleated erythroid cells are larger in aplastic anemia than in normal subjects (Bates and Bessman 1986). Further evidence of a qualitative stem cell change is the frequent increase in expression of the i antigen, hemoglobin F percentage, and in the number of hemoglobin F–containing cells in aplastic anemia (Bloom and Diamond 1968; Dover and Ogawa 1980). Both macrocytosis and hemoglobin F distinguish fetal from adult red cells. However, these two abnormal markers are not always expressed in the same cells, and macrocytosis appears to be the most uniformly expressed marker. Thus, the erythroid stem cells in aplastic anemia may reflect a partial reversion to fetal characteristics.

Despite the macrocytosis, the RDW in patients with aplastic anemia usually is normal if there has been no transfusion (fig. 2.19). Therefore, defective cell proliferation usually does not increase cellular heterogeneity, whether the erythropoiesis is microcytic or normocytic (anemia of chronic disease) or macrocytic (aplastic anemia). However, if the patient has been transfused, there will be two populations of cells, identifiable

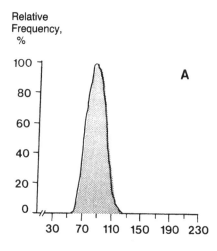

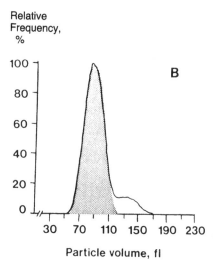

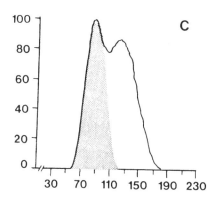

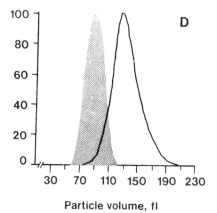

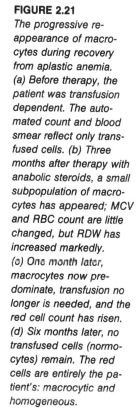

FIGURE 2.21
The progressive re-appearance of macro-cytes during recovery from aplastic anemia. (a) Before therapy, the patient was transfusion dependent. The auto-mated count and blood smear reflect only trans-fused cells. (b) Three months after therapy with anabolic steroids, a small subpopulation of macro-cytes has appeared; MCV and RBC count are little changed, but RDW has increased markedly. (c) One month later, macrocytes now pre-dominate, transfusion no longer is needed, and the red cell count has risen. (d) Six months later, no transfused cells (normo-cytes) remain. The red cells are entirely the pa-tient's: macrocytic and homogeneous.

by red cell volume histogram (fig. 2.20). Depending on the relative proportion of transfused cells, the MCV of the mixture will be within or above the normal range. RDW will be greatly increased. The histogram is especially useful to evaluate the patient who already has been transfused. The peripheral blood smear, MCV, and RDW may be confusing because of the transfusion. A distinct second population—the patient's own macrocytes—points to the correct diagnosis.

The red cell volume histogram is similarly useful in predicting recovery after patients have been treated—for example, with substituted steroids or antithymocyte globulin. Patients so treated usually have been transfused with red cells for so long and so frequently that both the MCV and the red cell histogram reflect only transfused red cells. In such cases, the MCV and RDW are normal until recovery begins. The initial sign of recovery is a reappearance of macrocytes as a separate peak in the histogram (Bessman and Gardner 1985). RDW simultaneously increases. Only later, when endogenous red cells are more numerous, does MCV become overtly above normal (fig. 2.21). Generally, the red cells remain macrocytic throughout the recovery, and in those patients whom we were able to follow for more than one year posttreatment, 15 of 17 remained macrocytic. The hemoglobin F–containing cells remained elevated in under half of those subjects studied. In 14 of 17 subjects, the RDW fell to normal when transfused red cells disappeared.

2.6.2 *Increased Heterogeneity*

2.6.2.1 Folate and Vitamin B_{12} Deficiency

Folic acid or vitamin B_{12} deficiency affects production of red cells, white cells, and platelets, but red cell changes are the ones that have been in the past most quantifiable and therefore

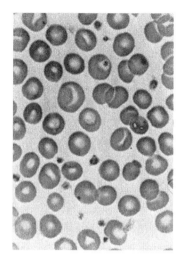

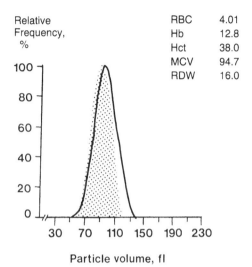

RBC	4.01
Hb	12.8
Hct	38.0
MCV	94.7
RDW	16.0

Particle volume, fl

FIGURE 2.22 *(above) Early folate deficiency. The MCV is still normal, and the red cell count is only slightly reduced, but the RDW already is clearly increased. Aniso- cytosis is the only abnor- mality on the blood smear.*

FIGURE 2.23 *(below) Severe folate deficiency. The red cell count is low, the MCV high, and the blood smear clearly abnormal. RDW is in- creased. As seen in the case of iron deficiency, the severe deficiency is easily diagnosed. This is a macrocytic hetero- geneous anemia.*

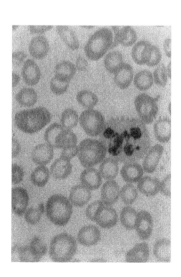

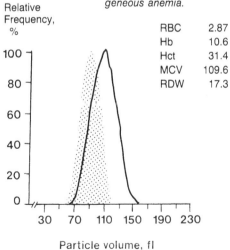

RBC	2.87
Hb	10.6
Hct	31.4
MCV	109.6
RDW	17.3

Particle volume, fl

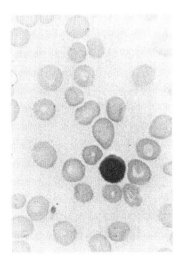

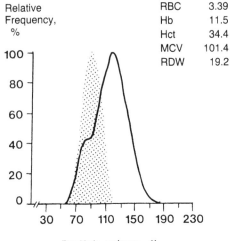

Particle volume, fl

FIGURE 2.24
Recovery from folate deficiency. The blood count was done ten days after therapy, during reticulocytosis. In this case the iron stores are normal, and the newly produced cells are visible as the small peak of cells in the normal range. RDW is higher than in untreated megaloblastic anemia because now two cell populations contribute to the heterogeneity.

most easily identified. The essential defect is a failure of DNA synthesis relative to RNA synthesis, and therefore a lag of nuclear maturation behind cytoplasmic maturation. Delayed nuclear maturation allows increased accumulation of cytoplasm before division. In the red cell series, this causes abnormally large cells. However, there is also an element of ineffective erythropoiesis. There is a rough correlation between the degree of anemia, the degree of macrocytosis, and the degree of ineffective erythropoiesis. Subjects with the most severe anemia and macrocytosis usually have marked hyperplasia in the bone marrow and bizarre nuclear morphology.

In a manner similar to that of iron deficiency, the heterogeneity of cell size changes before the MCV. The effect in megaloblastic disorders is that the red cell volume distribution increases before the MCV rises. Again, similar to iron deficiency, heterogeneity increases in proportion to the degree of anemia or macrocytosis (figs. 2.22 and 2.23). The peripheral blood smear shows the increase in heterogeneity and mean size.

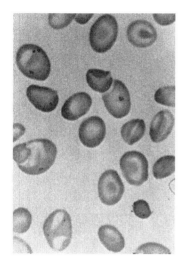

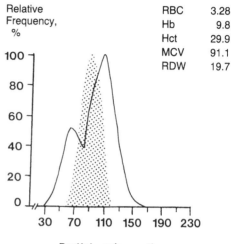

Relative Frequency, %

RBC	3.28
Hb	9.8
Hct	29.9
MCV	91.1
RDW	19.7

Particle volume, fl

FIGURE 2.25
Microcytic recovery from folate deficiency. Again two cell populations are clearly seen on the histogram: old macrocytes and newly produced microcytes. Concomitant iron deficiency has been unmasked. The RDW is markedly increased. The blood smear shows marked anisocytosis, but the viewer unaided by the histogram would have difficulty judging the size of the smaller cells. The MCV is normal, but only because it reflects the average of two abnormal populations. There is no population of red cells with a normal MCV.

During recovery from megaloblastic anemia, reticulocytosis follows therapy by four to five days. If there is only the megaloblastic deficiency, the reticulocytes and ensuing mature cells will be of normal size. In contrast, if there is also latent iron deficiency but only the folate or vitamin B_{12} deficiency is treated, the reticulocytes and ensuing mature red cells will be abnormally small (Bessman 1977*b*) (figs. 2.24 and 2.25). Such latent iron deficiency may not be detected by the initial MCV or RDW, since these will be abnormal whether there are two nutritional deficiencies or one. The ineffective erythropoiesis of megaloblastic nutritional deficiency tends to increase the amount of unutilized iron so that actual iron deficiency may be hidden by "normal" marrow iron staining or serum transferrin saturation. The size of the reticulocytes during therapy of megaloblastic anemia is an early clue to concomitant iron deficiency.

Severe megaloblastic anemia may cause such dyserythropoiesis that red cell fragmentation may appear in the peripheral blood. On the peripheral

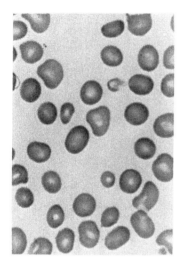

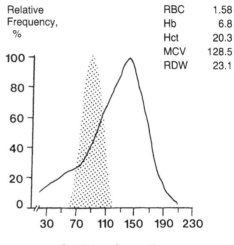

RBC	1.58
Hb	6.8
Hct	20.3
MCV	128.5
RDW	23.1

Particle volume, fl

FIGURE 2.26
Red cell fragmentation in megaloblastic anemia. The fragments form a plateau at all small sizes. Because the fragments are averaged with the intact cells, the MCV is less than that which would reflect whole cells only. The fragments disappear before reticulocytes reappear after therapy, and so the transient rise in MCV seen in such cases may reflect red cell fragment disappearance rather than reticulocytosis.

blood smear the fragments are easily detected. The red cell volume histogram will also show the population of fragments relatively distinct from whole macrocytes (fig. 2.26). The fragments, being smaller than the intact red cells in the same patient, will increase red cell heterogeneity but decrease the MCV. Thus, the degree of macrocytosis may seem relatively moderate in the face of marked anemia, but review of the histogram shows the true size of intact cells. When these patients recover, fragment production stops even before reticulocytosis and so MCV may transiently rise before it falls (Patel and Chanarin 1975).

2.6.2.2 Acquired Hemolytic Anemia

Acquired hemolytic anemia is associated with abnormalities of the blood count similar to those of hereditary hemolytic anemia. As long as the hemolysis is compensated to allow a normal hemoglobin, the reticulocyte count may be increased, but MCV and red cell volume heterogeneity (RDW) will be normal. If the hemolysis is a single occurrence—for example, in

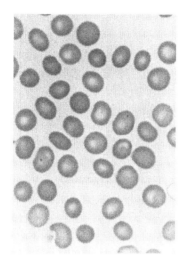

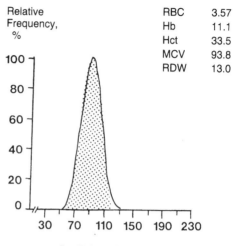

RBC	3.57
Hb	11.1
Hct	33.5
MCV	93.8
RDW	13.0

Particle volume, fl

FIGURE 2.27
*Acute transient hemolysis
with glucose-6-phosphate
dehydrogenase defi-
ciency (compare with fig.
2.19). The reticulocytes
are 12.6 percent. The red
cell count is reduced but
even when reticulocytosis
is marked, MCV and
RDW remain normal, to
produce a normocytic
homogeneous anemia.*

glucose-6-phosphate deficient subjects after
exposure to an oxidant drug—reticulocytes will
increase sharply after the acute hemolysis.
They will be only about 8 percent larger than the
mature cells, similar to the case in normal subjects or after acute hemorrhage (section 2.5.1.2)
(fig. 2.27). In proportion to the duration and
extent that anemia is produced by more chronic
acquired hemolysis, the MCV will rise. Such
hemolysis generally is autoimmune. It is thought
that the cause of the macrocytosis may be an
alteration in erythropoiesis, with a skipped division of the erythroid precursor leading to "stress"
erythropoiesis. Such "stress" presumably is
proportional to the degree of anemia (Williams
et al. 1983). The size of the mature cells parallels
the size of the reticulocyte and the degree of
anemia in human autoimmune hemolysis
(Bessman 1977*b*). Likewise, during recovery
MCV progressively falls as hemoglobin rises,
even though the reticulocyte count remains increased. This is further evidence that macrocytosis does not inevitably follow reticulocytosis,
but only reticulocytosis accompanied by altered

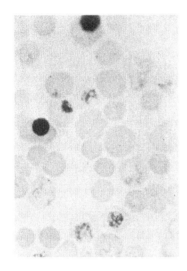

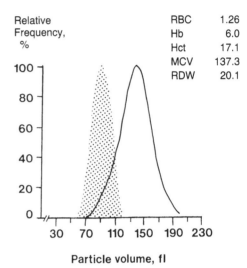

Particle volume, fl

FIGURE 2.28
Immune hemolytic ane-mia. At maximum hemo-lysis, reticulocytes are 37.1 percent and anemia is profound. Both MCV and RDW are increased, to make a macrocytic heterogeneous anemia. Nucleated red cells as well as reticulocytes (stained here to show the reticulin) are seen.

erythroid precursor maturation (figs. 2.28 and 2.29).

2.7 Artifacts

It should be emphasized that the abnormalities that are elicited by measurement techniques are in fact abnormalities of the blood, rather than measurement error. Indeed, the appearance of the following abnormal patterns should be strong clues to the responsible disorder. Recognition of these patterns is a major value of having the red cell histogram available for inspection (Cornbleet 1983). However, these artifacts will not identify all subjects with the disorders that cause them.

2.7.1 *Red Cell Fragmentation*

Red cell fragmentation may be caused by many factors, including:

malfunctioning cardiac prosthetic valve
sickle cell anemia
thrombotic thrombocytopenic purpura
hemolytic-uremic syndrome
disseminated intravascular coagulation
megaloblastic anemia (continued on p. 50)

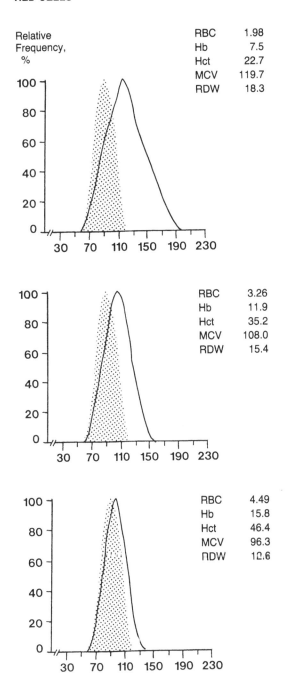

Relative
Frequency,
%

RBC	1.98
Hb	7.5
Hct	22.7
MCV	119.7
RDW	18.3

RBC	3.26
Hb	11.9
Hct	35.2
MCV	108.0
RDW	15.4

RBC	4.49
Hb	15.8
Hct	46.4
MCV	96.3
RDW	12.6

Particle volume, fl

FIGURE 2.29

Recovery from immune hemolytic anemia. During recovery, as the hemoglobin rises, the MCV falls. In all cases there is only a single peak of cells, and RDW is directly proportional to the degree of anemia. This shows how red cell heterogeneity parallels anemia in immune as well as non-immune hemolytic disorders.

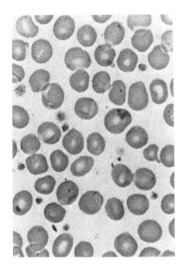

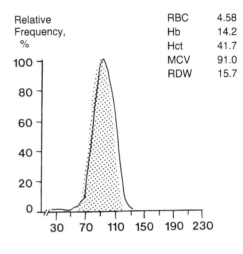

Relative
Frequency,
%

RBC	4.58
Hb	14.2
Hct	41.7
MCV	91.0
RDW	15.7

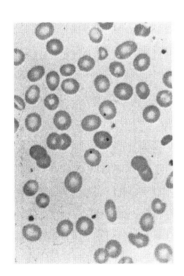

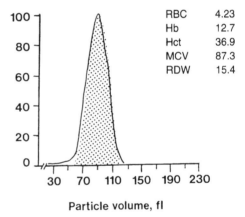

RBC	4.23
Hb	12.7
Hct	36.9
MCV	87.3
RDW	15.4

Particle volume, fl

FIGURE 2.30

Red cell fragmentation caused by burns. The MCV is normal in three of the four cases but the RDW is increased (normo- or microcytic heterogeneous indices). The histogram is pathognomonic for red cell fragmentation (compare fig. 2.26), here of normal-size cells. Without fragmentation there would be no plateau to the left side

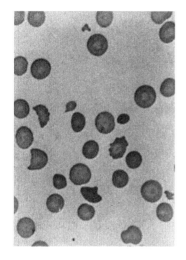

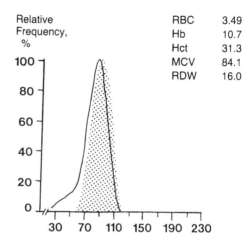

Relative Frequency, %	RBC	3.49
	Hb	10.7
	Hct	31.3
	MCV	84.1
	RDW	16.0

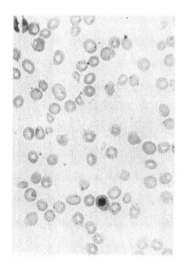

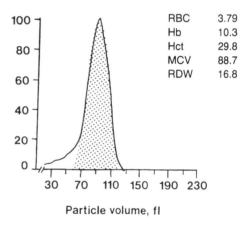

	RBC	3.79
	Hb	10.3
	Hct	29.8
	MCV	88.7
	RDW	16.8

Particle volume, fl

of the peak. The reader should consider how few fragments could be determined reproducibly from the blood smear without prior clinical information, versus the objective abnormality seen on the histogram.

burns
metastatic tumor
cytotoxic chemotherapy

Careful examination of the peripheral blood smear will reveal the fragments. Detection is aided by the red cell histogram, which will reveal the fragments when they equal about 0.8 percent of total cells (the equivalent of one per high-power field). In such cases, the peak of intact cells is joined by a skew or plateau of smaller fragments (fig. 2.30). In extreme circumstances, the fragments are so numerous that not only is the histogram altered but the MCV is lowered and RDW is increased as well (Bessman 1977c). More often, the MCV is within the normal range, but the abnormal histogram is a clear clue. Those fragments <36 fl are not counted as red cells and so RBC and hematocrit are artifactually low. Because the hemoglobin measurement remains accurate (with severe fragmentation free plasma hemoglobin will be included also), in extreme cases the MCHC is artifactually high. In contrast, we have found that examination of the peripheral smear without prior knowledge of the disorder identifies red cell fragments reliably only when they exceed 2 percent of cells.

2.7.2 Lymphocytes

When whole blood is analyzed, cells are defined by criteria different from those of traditional morphology. Red cells are no longer defined by their hemoglobin pigment, but by nominal volume. If other cells also fall within the criteria defining red cell volume, such cells are counted as red cells. Mature lymphocytes may have a nominal mean Coulter volume as low as 180 fl, with the smallest cells being 150 fl. The average value for lymphocytes is 220 fl. However, even if all such lymphocytes were counted as red cells, in normal subjects the ratio of lymphocytes to red cells

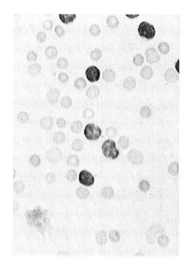

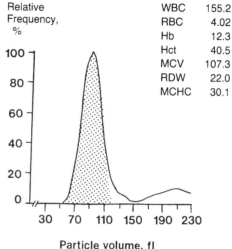

Particle volume, fl

FIGURE 2.31
Chronic lymphocytic leu-
kemia. The lymphocyte
count is markedly ele-
vated, sufficient to cause
a clear second population
with a peak at 209 fl,
which is counted as "red
cells." Therefore, MCV
and RDW are increased,
but MCHC falls.

is so small that the error caused by inclusion of lymphocytes is small.

Normal cell count values:

$$\frac{(8 \times 10^9 \text{ white cells/l}) \ (40\% \text{ lymphocytes})}{5 \times 10^{12} \text{ red cells/l}} = \frac{1}{1500}$$

In chronic lymphocytic leukemia, the white count may rise to $150 \times 10^9/l$ or more, and be virtually all lymphocytes. Modest anemia with a RBC count reduced to $3 \times 10^{12}/l$ is common. In this situation, lymphocytes are 5 percent as numerous as red cells, and so the MCV is spuriously increased by 5 percent of the difference botwoon rod colls and lymphocytos (o.g., lymphocyte mean volume of 220 fl; 5 percent of 220–90 fl, or about 6 fl). The MCH and MCHC are proportionately spuriously low, because the lymphocytes are counted as red cells but contain no hemoglobin. The artifactual inclusion is identified easily by the red cell volume histogram, because lymphocytes are larger than red cell doublets (see below) and macrocytes rarely exceed 145 fl (fig. 2.31).

Granulocytes, in contrast, are so much larger that they do not similarly compromise the red cell indices. However, if the white cell count exceeds $200 \times 10^9/l$, the hemoglobin value may be altered by the turbidity caused by granulocytes. A spurious Hb value will also affect the MCH and MCHC.

2.7.3 Red Cell Agglutinins

Agglutinins cause single red cells to clump together. Depending on the nature of the agglutinin, the temperature at which it can agglutinate red cells (thermal amplitude) may approach 37°C or be only at a substantially lower temperature. The former can cause agglutination within the vessels of distal fingers, toes, ears, etc., in which the blood flow is cooled even slightly. In contrast, the latter occurs only as a laboratory abnormality. Both, however, may signal an underlying immunologic disorder such as lymphoma (Pruzanski and Shumak 1977). In the past some instruments briefly were modified to warm the diluent and eliminate the cold-agglutinin "artifact." However, this approach obscures the important clinical information and is no longer used. While low-thermal-amplitude cold agglutinins do not cause in vivo damage, they are not simply reflections of erratic tech-

TABLE 2.7 Changes in Red Cell Indices Caused by Cold Agglutinins

Item	At 20°C	At 37°C
RBC ($10^{12}/l$)	2.97	3.75
MCV (fl)	103.0	91.0
Hct (%)	31.0	34.0
Hb (g/dl)	11.2	11.2
MCHC (%)	36.1	33.3

Note: The same blood sample is shown: once, at room temperature, and once at body temperature. See the text for the cause of the changes.

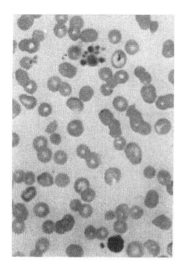

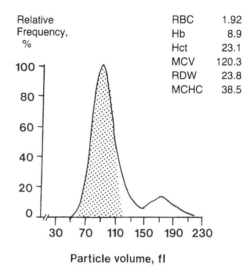

RBC	1.92
Hb	8.9
Hct	23.1
MCV	120.3
RDW	23.8
MCHC	38.5

Relative Frequency, %

Particle volume, fl

FIGURE 2.32
Red cell cold agglutinins. The red cell count is reduced but hemoglobin is accurate. The MCV is increased because it includes the doublets with a mean of 165 fl. In this case the agglutination is seen on the blood smear, but in many cases only the in vitro conditions of the counter will elicit the biological abnormality.

nology. Rather, processing in an automated counter elicits an otherwise latent biologic abnormality. This allows investigation of the cause of the abnormal agglutinin in over twice the number of cases (in our experience) that would come to light if clinical signs and symptoms alone were the means of detection.

In the dilute blood suspension used by most automated counters, agglutination will be predominantly as red cell doublets, rather than the larger clumps seen on the peripheral smear (fig. 2.32). One might expect that such doublets would be twice the size of single red cells. However, particularly in impedance counters, doublet cells offer about 180 percent of the impedance of single cells. In large part this is because of the altered shape and deformability of a doublet (Bessman 1980b). A typical example is shown in figure 2.32. The single red cells are 91 fl, and the doublets are 165 fl: doublets measured 10 percent less than the sum of their parts. The apparent fall in red cell count caused by clumping, therefore, is not quite matched by a rise in MCV. As a result the product of red cell count and

MCV (the hematocrit) is artifactually reduced. Because hemoglobin measurement is not affected by agglutination, the ratio of Hb/Hct, or MCHC, rises. This abnormality is well documented with cold agglutinins (Brittin et al. 1969; Hattersley et al. 1971; Petrucci et al. 1971; Solanki and Blackburn 1985), and in two cases of warm agglutinins (Weiss and Bessman 1984). Our experience in a warm climate is that cold agglutinins are a more common cause for high MCHC than is hereditary spherocytosis. The best clue is that the mode of the RBC histogram does not match the reported MCV. The effect of cold agglutinins usually is reversible in vitro by warming the whole or diluted blood above the temperature of the agglutinin's thermal amplitude (see table 2.7).

It is possible that macroglobulins, cryoglobulins, or rouleau formation could cause similar artifactual results, but such cases have not been reported.

2.7.4 Osmotic Changes

Water flows along a gradient across cell membranes far faster than osmotically active solutes such as glucose. Red cells "loaded" with glucose in a hyperglycemic subject then are hypertonic in relation to the nominally isotonic diluent used in automated counters. Therefore, hyperglycemia allows an artifactual change in MCV by the following mechanism. Water from the diluent flows into the red cells far more rapidly than glucose can flow out, so the red cell's initial osmotic equilibration is achieved by net red cell swelling. Because the red cells are exposed to diluent for only a few seconds before being measured, there is no chance for further equilibration to correct the swelling. This artifact may cause serious overstatement of the red cell size (Beautyman and Bills 1982). Here the rest of the automated count is crucial. Red cell count and hemoglobin are accurate. Therefore, the hematocrit is spuriously high, MCH is correct, and MCHC is

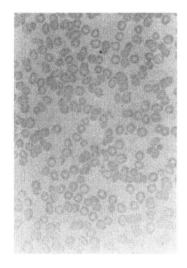

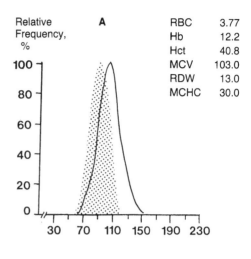

	A		
		RBC	3.77
		Hb	12.2
		Hct	40.8
		MCV	103.0
		RDW	13.0
		MCHC	30.0

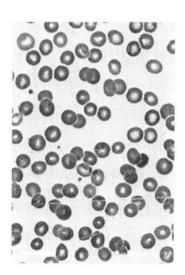

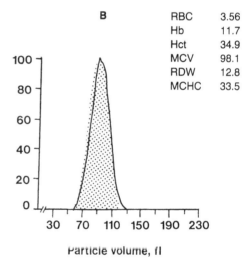

	B		
		RBC	3.56
		Hb	11.7
		Hct	34.9
		MCV	98.1
		RDW	12.8
		MCHC	33.5

Particle volume, fl

FIGURE 2.33

Osmotic changes caused by hyperglycemia. (a) The blood sugar is 883 mg/dl: whereas the MCV is increased, RDW remains normal because all cells swell proportionately. (b) After the blood sugar falls to normal, so does the MCV.

TABLE 2.8 Abnormalities Caused by Artifacts

Item	RBC	Hb	Hct	MCV	MCH	MCHC	Artifact Appears on Histogram at
Red cell fragmentation	↓	↑	↓	↓	↑	↑	< 80 fl
Lymphocytes	↑	N	↑	↑	↓	↓	>180 fl
Red cell agglutination	↓	N	↓	↑	↑	↑	150–170 fl
Hyperglycemia	N	N	↑	↑	N	↓	—
Free plasma hemoglobin	N	↑	N	N	↑	↑	—

spuriously low, in linear proportion to the amount of spurious macrocytosis (fig. 2.33). Because all red cells are affected equally, the RDW does not change during the hyperglycemia-induced macrocytosis (unpublished data).

The artifacts discussed in these four sections (2.7.1–2.7.4) are summarized in table 2.8.

3
Platelets

3.1 Introduction: The Biologic Determinants of Platelet Size

Platelets, the fragmentation product of mega-karyocytes, are enucleate, but have an active enzymology and physiology. They are much more variable in size than are other blood cells, nearly tenfold from largest to smallest, in contrast to the twofold range of red cells. Several hypotheses have been offered to explain this remarkable range of size:

Shrinkage with age. This is a controversial hypothesis. Some researchers have shown that on an average, the oldest platelets are the smallest (Karpatkin 1978; Garg et al. 1971); others deny this shrinkage (Mezzano et al. 1981; Thompson et al. 1983*b*, 1983*c*). Additional data bearing on this point are discussed later.

Heterogeneity of megakaryocyte fragmentation. This, too, is controversial. Within a single megakaryocyte, several thousand cytoplasmic portions are formed into platelets (Tavassoli 1980). Electron microscopy of mature megakaryocytes shows that the portions of cytoplasm that become platelets seem to (by a two-dimensional representation of a three-dimensional process) vary within a single megakaryocyte (Paulus et al. 1979, 1983).

Heterogeneity of megakaryocytes. Megakaryocytes normally occur in several classes of DNA content, or ploidy (Penington et al. 1976). Higher-ploidy megakaryocytes have been asso-

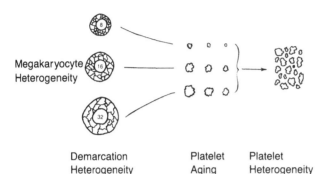

Megakaryocyte
Heterogeneity

Demarcation   Platelet   Platelet
Heterogeneity   Aging   Heterogeneity

FIGURE 3.1
*Causes of heterogeneity
of platelet size. Each
megakaryocyte has an
intrinsic variation in the
size of platelets it forms:
higher-ploidy mega-
karyocytes produce larger
platelets than do lower-
ploidy megakaryocytes;
and platelets shrink to
some degree in the
circulation.*

ciated with larger platelets, and so it is further
proposed that each megakaryocyte ploidy class
may be associated with a specific platelet size
(Penington et al. 1976; Bessman 1984). One
group has speculated that larger megakaryocytes are associated with an increased
heterogeneity of their platelet progeny (Paulus et
al. 1983) but this remains to be proved. Levine
et al. (1982) have shown that higher-ploidy
megakaryocytes are larger. It remains uncertain
whether the number of platelets formed per
megakaryocyte is independent of ploidy.

Because there is substantial evidence for each
of these hypotheses, it is probable that all three
contribute to the final substantial heterogeneity
of platelet size in the normal subject (fig. 3.1).

Platelet size is distributed in a nearly log-
normal manner (fig. 3.2) (Paulus et al. 1979; Dighiero et al. 1981). The distribution histogram is
valuable in that it is this shape as long as only
platelets are being measured. The histogram de-
viates progressively from log-normal to the extent that there are artifacts (see section 3.9).
From the distribution histogram the integrated
mean volume can be calculated as mean platelet
volume (MPV) (Mayer, Chin, and Baistey 1985;
Bessman, Williams, and Gilmer 1981). Platelet
volume heterogeneity has been calculated: in

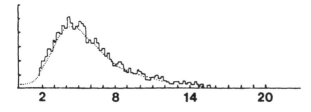

2   8   14   20

FIGURE 3.2
Distribution of platelet size. Although the distribution is not precisely log-normal, it is sufficiently close that log-normal analysis can be used. The scale of volume is in femtoliters (fl), but is only nominal, and in standard Coulter calibration this scale does not indicate actual particle (platelet) size. Two histograms are shown: the actual data (solid line) and the best-fit log-normal distribution from which the platelet variables are calculated.

one instrument (Coulter Counter Model S-Plus series) the geometric standard deviation is the basis of the "platelet distribution width" (PDW) (Bessman, Williams, and Gilmer 1982). The clinical use of PDW remains to be determined.

3.2 Normal Values

For most hematologic values there is a single range of values that includes and defines normal subjects. For instance, a normal range of hemoglobin and hematocrit has been defined (depending on age and sex). Likewise, there is a normal range of MCV and red cell count. For platelets, there are only two variables that are routinely measured—platelet count and mean platelet volume. There is a single normal range for platelet count. However, the situation is more complex for MPV: platelet count and MPV are inversely but nonlinearly related (Garg et al. 1971; Bessman, Williams, and Gilmer 1981). Figure 3.3 and table 3.1 show this relation among 683 medical, nursing, and allied health students (Bessman, Williams, and Gilmer 1981). This relation is confirmed in several other studies (Giles 1981; Rowan and Fraser 1982). Furthermore, it is not an artifact of automated counters: visual micrometry of platelet size confirms the relation (Ziegler, Murphy, and Gardner 1978). Note that the relation does not form a straight line—the mean value for MPV changes less and less as platelet count rises. This means that the "platelet-crit," the product of platelet count and size analogous to the hematocrit, is not constant

MPV, fl

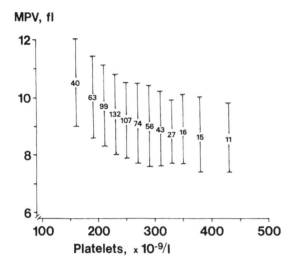

Platelets, $\times 10^{-9}/l$

FIGURE 3.3
Platelet count and size (MPV) in 683 normal subjects aged 20–34 years. There is no difference between male and female; or among white, Mexican-American, or black. The subjects are stratified by platelet count: for each subgroup, the number shows how many subjects were in the group and the mean MPV for that range of platelet count. The bars show 2 SD about the mean. Source: Bessman, Williams, and Gilmer 1981.

along the range of normals. From the data in figure 3.3 and table 3.1:

Normal subjects with $150 \times 10^9/l$ platelets have an average MPV of 10.6 fl, so platelet-crit (platelet count $\times$ MPV) is 0.159. Normal subjects with $400 \times 10^9/l$ platelets have an average MPV of 8.5 fl, so platelet-crit is 0.360.

This wide variation in platelet-crit among normal subjects suggests two things. First, it is not helpful to use platelet-crit as a variable to determine normal or abnormal platelet results. "Normal" values depend on the platelet count. A "constant" platelet-crit cannot be obtained by log transformation of either or both variables. Second, because platelet-crit is not a constant among individuals, or as shown later, in a given individual, platelet-crit is unlikely to be an important physiological regulator. Hemoglobin level, in contrast, is constant among normal subjects, and any change from baseline has a potent feedback to modulate erythropoiesis. To judge whether an individual's platelet values are normal, MPV and platelet count both should be related to a nomo-

TABLE 3.1 Normal Numerical Values for Platelet Size at Various Normal Platelet Counts

		Platelet Count $\times 10^9/l$											
		160	190	210	230	250	270	290	310	330	350	380	430
Statistical	160	—	NS	0.05	0.01	0.01	0.01	0.01	0.01	0.01	0.01	0.01	0.01
difference	190		—	NS	NS	0.05	0.02	0.02	0.01	0.01	0.01	0.01	0.01
($P <$ ___)	210			—	NS	NS	0.05	0.02	0.02	0.01	0.01	0.01	0.01
from mean	230				—	NS	NS	0.05	0.02	0.01	0.01	0.01	0.01
value for MPV	250					—	NS	NS	NS	0.02	0.05	0.02	0.01
in patients with	270						—	NS	NS	0.05	NS	0.05	0.02
platelets of	290							—	NS	NS	NS	0.05	0.02
($\times 10^9/l$)	310								—	NS	NS	NS	0.05
	330									—	NS	NS	NS
	350										—	NS	NS
	380											—	NS

Source: Bessman, Williams, and Gilmer 1981.

gram similar to that shown in figure 3.3. This nomogram now is part of the printout of some Coulter instruments. If the two-dimensional plot of MPV and platelet count falls more than the technological error away from the mean $\pm$ 2 SD, the patient's platelets are abnormal in MPV, whatever the count.

These data are derived with a particular technology: this nomogram has been satisfactory for other laboratories with the same technology. With other machines and calibrators, the *scale* of MPV will differ, but the shape of the nomogram will be the same (Giles 1981; Rowan and Fraser 1082). Thoroforo, oach laboratory should use a nomogram appropriate to its technology.

In fact, red cell count and MCV similarly do not actually have independent normal ranges. What is held constant in normal subjects is hematocrit (or hemoglobin), and so even within the "normal" range those subjects with the highest red cell counts have the lowest MCV, and vice versa (table 3.2). It is by convention that the entire range among normal subjects is given, but

TABLE 3.2 MCV in 500 Normal Male Subjects with Various Red Cell Counts

RBC	MCV
4.70–4.90	93.9±5.0
4.90–5.10	91.8±5.7
5.10–5.30	90.0±5.6
5.30–5.50	86.3±6.1
5.50–5.70	83.8±3.2

Note: As discussed in the text, there is not a constant "normal" range for either value.

certain combinations are incompatible with normality. For instance, MCV of 82 fl and red cell count of $4.75 \times 10^{12}/l$ each are "normal" per se, but taken together would be associated with anemia for males (hematocrit of 38.9 percent). The definition of "normal" cell size as a function of cell count is simply more apparent in platelets than in red cells. There is as yet no described attribute of the platelet that is analogous to the physiologic constant of hemoglobin or hematocrit for the red cell.

Platelet morphology is particularly treacherous for estimation of platelet size. Although painstaking quantitation of platelet diameters from a blood smear by eyepiece micrometer is quite accurate (Ziegler, Murphy, and Gardner 1978), a subjective impression without quantitation may give a false impression. "Giant" platelets often are considered suggestive of congenital, myeloproliferative, or hyperdestructive disorders. However, large platelets draw more attention than do small ones, and so frequently a slide is read as showing unquantitated "giant platelets." Because of the broad distribution of platelet size, even when the *mean* value is reduced, the largest 5 or 10 percent will be "large." These largest forms will be especially noticeable in patients with thrombocytosis, even though the mean value is reduced (fig. 3.4). For these

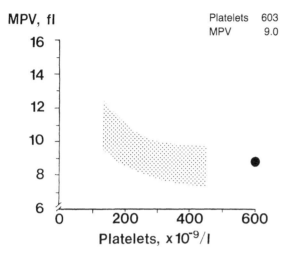

MPV, fl

Platelets   603
MPV   9.0

Platelets, x 10⁻⁹/l

FIGURE 3.4

Thrombocytosis. Although the MPV is normal, when there are so many platelets a few will be at the large end of the spectrum. Because these are the most noticeable on the blood smear, undue significance may be given to them. In this and the following examples, the dot will plot a representative case's platelet count and MPV that are shown at the top. The range of all patients in the particular disease group also will be outlined against the nomogram of values in normal subjects (shaded area).

reasons the simple presence of large platelets is rather nonspecific. However, it is important to visually examine the peripheral blood smear to assure against artifacts and to detect the occasional cell that is abnormal or exceptional.

Disorders of platelets that are first detectable from the automated blood count can be grouped into the five categories shown in figure 3.5:

    normal platelet count and MPV
    high MPV, low platelet count
    high platelet count, normal MPV
    inappropriately high MPV
    inappropriately low MPV

Using this classification, 8 percent of inpatients in a tertiary hospital had abnormal values, with as many having abnormal MPV with normal count as had an abnormal platelet count (Bessman 1985). Because those patients with abnormal MPV all had an identifiable hematologic disorder, addition of MPV allows twice the detection of abnormalities that platelet count does alone. Note that the classification of anemias was well detailed with a sound physiologic basis long before automated counts. Even so, additional variables available with the new tech-

MPV, fl

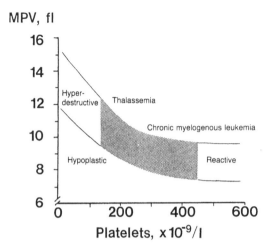

FIGURE 3.5
Classification of platelet disorders.

Platelets, x 10⁻⁹/l

nology identified new disorders (e.g., early iron deficiency). In contrast, classification of platelet disorders is much less detailed, and the newly available automated MPV may be an important identifier of new disorders.

Anticoagulants affect platelet size. EDTA, which is the usual anticoagulant for the routine blood count (purple-top tube), alters platelet shape, from disc to sphere. This shape change causes an approximate 20 percent increase in apparent MPV in the first two hours after exposure to EDTA (Bull and Zucker 1965; Mundschenk et al. 1976). The change can be minimized by inclusion of ACD anticoagulant (Thompson et al. 1983a). However, the change in MPV is equally present in large and small platelets, and so the same distinctions that are made before EDTA exposure are equally valid after (Levin and Bessman 1983). Therefore, while the presence of an artifact should be recognized (Threatte et al. 1984) the use of EDTA anticoagulant does not appear to affect the classification of platelet disorders by platelet size, or use of this for understanding of megakaryocyte physiology.

The following chapter suggests how use of

TABLE 3.3 The Morphophysiologic Classification of Platelet Disorders

	Platelet Count		
MPV	Low	Normal	High
Abnormally low in hypoproliferative and megaloblastic disorders	Aplastic anemia; megaloblastic disorders; cytotoxic chemotherapy	Same disorders	
Appropriate to count in hyperdestructive/ hyperproductive disorders	ITP eclampsia	Normal	Reactive thrombocytosis
Abnormal size in hereditary and myeloproliferative disorders	High MPV Bernard-Soulier Low MPV Wiskott-Aldrich	High MPV Thalassemia Myelofibrosis Myelodysplasia	High MPV Chronic myelogenous leukemia
Changes with abnormal splenic function	Hypersplenism (low MPV)		Splenectomy (high MPV)

MPV can improve the description of platelet disorders from the automated blood count. Even diseases that often are associated with abnormal values have enough variability that individual patients may have normal values. All patients with a given disease cannot be detected by the automated blood count: rather, those subjects with abnormal values should be studied further. Table 3.3 shows how use of the platelet count and MPV allow a classification of platelet disorders that is based on morphology but illustrates the physiology of platelet production.

3.3 Diseases with Normal Platelet Values

Diabetes and atherosclerotic coronary vascular disease are suspected to include a certain degree of abnormal platelet function. Chronic lymphocytic leukemia is a clonal abnormality of lymphocytes that spares the megakaryocyte line.

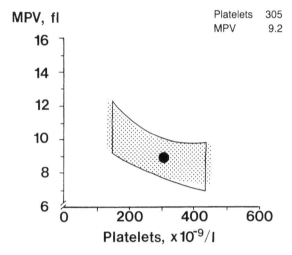

MPV, fl

Platelets   305
MPV   9.2

FIGURE 3.6

Platelet indices in 73 patients with atherosclerotic heart disease. For any given platelet count, MPV has essentially the same range as in normal subjects.

Schizophrenia is associated with abnormal monoamine oxidase levels. Monoamine oxidase also is found in platelets, raising the question of whether schizophrenia is associated with a platelet disorder. Because each of these disorders might be considered to have a possible platelet abnormality, we measured platelet size and count in groups of such patients. Each of these disorders was associated with normal platelet size and count (Bessman, Williams, and Gilmer 1982). Figure 3.6 summarizes data in atherosclerotic patients; MPV was essentially the same in the other two diseases. Increases in MPV that were reported to be associated with acute myocardial infarction (Cameron et al. 1983; Sewell et al. 1984) were associated with decreases in platelet count as well: at any given platelet count, the MPV was the same as in normal subjects (Van der Lelie and Brakenhoff 1983). These changes suggest an acute thrombolytic process with marrow compensation, rather than an intrinsic platelet abnormality.

3.4 High Platelet Count, Normal MPV

Reactive thrombocytosis accompanies a broad range of inflammatory, infectious, nutritional, and

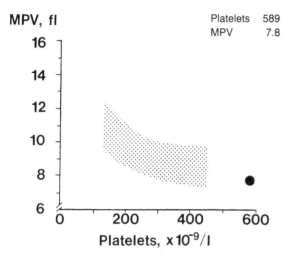

MPV, fl

Platelets 589
MPV 7.8

FIGURE 3.7
Reactive thrombocytosis. In patients with inflammatory, infectious, or neoplastic causes of thrombocytosis, MPV is on average below that of normals. MPV appears to reach an asymptotic low value at about 500 x 10⁹/l. The relation of high platelet count to low MPV tends to continue the shape of the nonlinear inverse relation of MPV to platelet count seen in normals.

neoplastic dieases (Levin and Conley 1964), with platelet counts rising as high as $1.5 \times 10^{12}/l$. The magnitude of thrombocytosis does not correlate well with the severity of the primary disease. The cause of the reactive thrombocytosis in unclear, because the disorders described above do not appear to have a common effect upon the bone marrow. In reactive thrombocytosis, MPV tends to be smaller than the MPV associated with high-normal platelet counts in normal subjects (fig. 3.7) (Friedhoff et al. 1978; Levin and Bessman 1983; Robbins and Barnard 1983). As is discussed above, on the peripheral blood smear, despite the low MPV, the large platelets stand out among the far more numerous small platelets.

3.5 Low Platelet Count, High MPV

Subjects with immune thrombocytopenic purpura (ITP) have increased peripheral blood platelet destruction, increased platelet production, increased MPV, and decreased platelet count (fig. 3.8) (Garg, Lackner, and Karpatkin 1971). Among individuals recovering from ITP, and among subjects with chronic ITP with various degrees of compensation, MPV has an inverse, nonlinear

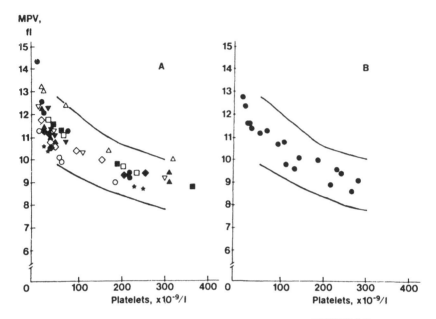

MPV,
fl

A

B

Platelets, x10^{-9}/l

Platelets, x10^{-9}/l

FIGURE 3.8
Immune thrombocyto-penia. (a) MPV during the course of recovery from acute ITP (aggregate data in 11 cases). (b) MPV in 17 subjects with stable chronic ITP at various levels of compensation (adapted from Levin and Bessman 1983). The values continue the inverse nonlinear relation of MPV and platelet count in normal subjects. When platelet count is normal in ITP, so is MPV.

relation with platelet count that continues the inverse, nonlinear relation seen in normal subjects (Levin and Bessman 1983; Garg, Amorosi, and Karpatkin 1971; Bessman 1982). Similarly a high MPV is seen in cases of thrombocytopenia attributable to other causes of increased peripheral destruction such as preeclampsia (Giles 1982; Giles and Inglis 1981; Fay et al. 1983) and systemic lupus erythematosus. Thus, when the bone marrow is intrinsically normal but is responding to the stimulus of thrombocytopenia caused by peripheral platelet destruction, MPV is high. In these cases the DNA content (ploidy) and size of megakaryocytes also are increased, as are the more primitive megakaryocyte progenitors (Ebbe et al. 1968; Penington et al. 1976; Levin et al. 1982; Bessman 1984). Also, a high MPV is seen in patients during the first stages of recovery from thrombocytopenia caused by bone marrow suppression. Here, too, the bone marrow *during recovery* is intrinsically

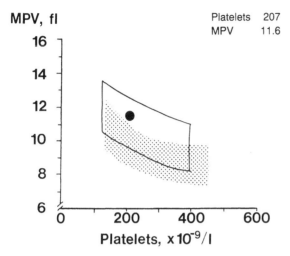

MPV, fl

| Platelets | 207 |
| MPV | 11.6 |

FIGURE 3.9

Heterozygous thalas-semia. The mean tends to be above normal at any platelet count, but the bio-logical scatter is such that only about half of the sub-jects with heterozygous thalassemia have MPV outside the normal range. The platelets may appear especially large against the backdrop of small red cells.

normal, responding to peripheral thrombo-cytopenia, and accompanied by increased megakaryocyte ploidy (Bessman 1982).

In contrast, rapid platelet turnover alone does not cause high MPV. In subjects with ITP com-pensated sufficiently to allow a low-normal platelet count, MPV is equal to that in normal subjects with similar platelet counts (Levin and Bessman 1983). This relation of individual cell size to peripheral-blood mass of the cell type is similar to hemolytic anemia: only when the peripheral counts are low does the cell size increase.

3.6 Inappropriately High MPV

Approximately half of subjects with heterozygous α- or β-thalassemia have above normal MPV but normal platelet count. This is true whether the subjects are of black, Mediterranean, southeast Asian, or nominally Northern European descent (Levin and Bessman 1983) (fig. 3.9). The dis-tribution histograms show that red cell fragments are not present to be confused with platelets (compare fig. 3.18). The biologic cause of the high MPV is unknown. Interestingly, there are at least four distinct hematologic alterations in het-

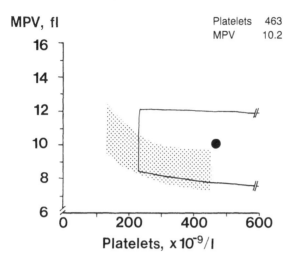

FIGURE 3.10

Chronic myelogenous leukemia. Most patients, even those with normal platelet counts, have abnormally high MPV.

erozygous thalassemia: altered globin chain synthesis, altered red cell size, altered platelet size, and altered resistance to malarial invasion. Only part of the molecular pathology is known.

Other causes of high MPV include chronic myelogenous leukemia, myelofibrosis, and splenectomy. Chronic myelogenous leukemia and myelofibrosis are generalized myeloproliferative disorders, and in both the platelets often, although not always, are large and abnormally heterogeneous (fig. 3.10) (Vainchenker et al. 1979; Holme et al. 1982; Bessman, Williams, and Gilmer 1982). In these disorders there are truly "giant" platelets in the peripheral blood smear. In contrast, in our experience and others' (Small and Bettigole 1981), myeloproliferative disorders such as essential thrombocythemia and polycythemia vera are not associated with abnormally large platelets. In these disorders, the bone marrow is hyperproliferative but the resulting cells are phenotypically normal (fig. 3.11).

After splenectomy for any reason, a different mechanism affects platelet size. The "filtering" function of the spleen is lost. It is postulated that the spleen preferentially sequesters the larger

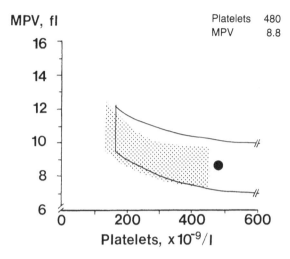

MPV, fl

Platelets 480
MPV 8.8

Platelets, x 10⁻⁹/ l

FIGURE 3.11
Polycythemia vera. The platelet values are congruent with normal values or those of reactive thrombocytosis unless there is also iron deficiency. About 20 percent of subjects iron-deficient for any reason have high MPV.

platelets within a given subject's peripheral platelet population. However, after splenectomy the feedback from the peripheral-blood platelets to thrombopoiesis in the marrow apparently changes, for thrombocytosis and increased MPV often persist permanently. Perhaps the largest group of such patients is adults with hemoglobin SS, who are functionally asplenic. The high MPV in these patients (Freedman and Karpatkin 1975; Holme et al. 1982) presumably is due to the asplenia rather than associated with the hemoglobinopathy per se. In our five patients with posttraumatic splenectomy, MPV was similarly increased for the high-normal platelet count.

The rare hereditary platelet disorder, Bernard-Soulier disease, is associated with exceptionally large platelets and moderate-to-severe thrombocytopenia (Gralnick et al. 1982). Certain other uncommon hereditary disorders such as Epstein's syndrome (Epstein et al. 1972) and the grey-platelet syndrome (White 1979) are similar (Gardner and Bessman 1983; Howard, Hutton, and Hardisty 1981). Like the myeloproliferative disorders, these disorders probably include an intrinsic megakaryocyte defect.

An occasional patient with reactive thrombo-

cytosis and a substantial minority of iron deficient subjects have increased MPV (Levin and
Bessman 1983; Karpatkin, Garg, and Freedman
1974). The connection between iron and thrombopoiesis remains unclear because bleeding, as
well as the underlying lesion causing blood loss,
promotes thrombocytosis.

In this and the next section, abnormalities of
platelet size (MPV) are shown often in subjects
with normal platelet counts. In most of these, the
range of MPV is shifted up or down, but there
remains a substantial overlap with normal values
in many cases of heterozygous thalassemia, iron
deficiency, chronic myelogenous leukemia, or
folate deficiency. Abnormal MPV simply suggests consideration of the possibilities listed.
Subjects with abnormal MPV values and no apparent other hematologic abnormality may have
an as-yet uncharacterized disorder, but this is
not clearly shown.

3.7 Inappropriately Low MPV

A different group of disorders are associated
with an MPV lower than that found in normal
subjects or in hyperdestructive thrombocytopenia. Disorders with low MPV generally
are those of marrow suppression: they include
myelotoxic chemotherapy, aplastic anemia, and
septic thrombocytopenia (Roper et al. 1977;
Bessman, Williams, and Gilmer 1982). Although
there still may remain the occasional large platelet as the extreme of the distribution (fig. 3.12),
the average size is reduced. Note that the MPV
is approximately the same as is found in reactive
thrombocytosis. However, in the myelosuppres-
sive disorders listed, the same low MPV is found
with a much lower platelet count. Therefore, the
relation of MPV and platelet count is markedly
divergent from the continuum formed by hyperdestructive thrombocytopenia-normal-reactive
thrombocytosis. In aplastic anemia, even when
the platelet count is in the normal range, MPV

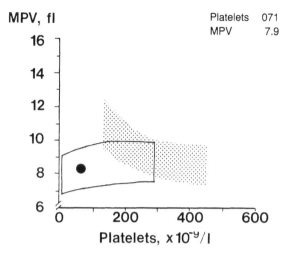

MPV, fl

Platelets 071
MPV 7.9

Platelets, x 10⁻⁹/l

FIGURE 3.12
Aplastic anemia. The MPV is subnormal, even when the platelet count is normal. The deficiency of the MPV is especially striking in thrombocytopenic subjects in contrast to subjects equally thrombocytopenic from immune causes (fig. 3.8).

frequently is abnormally low, although the divergence from normal is not so pronounced (fig. 3.12). This appears to be a permanent marker, as is increased red cell size, of the stem cell defect that remains even when the cell counts return to normal (Bessman and Gardner 1984). In isolated megakaryocyte hypoplasia, MPV also is abnormally small for the low platelet count (Stoll et al. 1981).

MPV also is reduced in megaloblastic anemia, whether caused by folate or vitamin B_{12} deficiency, or cytotoxic chemotherapy (Bessman, Williams, and Gilmer 1982). This abnormality again is most apparent at lower platelet counts, because the same MPV is increasingly divergent from the values caused by hyperdestruction at lower platelet counts (fig. 3.13). As with aplastic anemia, even subjects with normal platelet counts have, on average, low MPV. However, not all such cases have clearly abnormal MPV, just as all do not have clearly increased red cell size. The defective MPV is corrected within two weeks after specific treatment of the deficiency (Dzik 1982). As noted in section 3.5, hyperdestructive anemia or thrombocytopenia are marked by increases in the affected cells' size. It

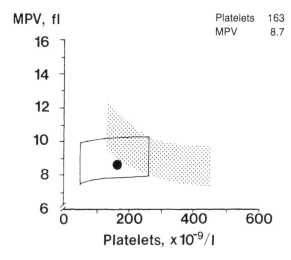

MPV, fl

Platelets 163
MPV 8.7

FIGURE 3.13
*Megaloblastic anemia.
The MPV is low at any
platelet count. As in
aplastic anemia, the in-
verse relation makes the
abnormality especially
apparent in thrombo-
cytopenic subjects, but
there remains a defect in
MPV even when the
platelet count is low-
normal.*

may seem paradoxical that megaloblastic red
cells and white cells are abnormally large,
whereas megaloblastic platelets are small. However, both abnormalities reflect the defective
DNA synthesis. Platelet size is directly proportional to megakaryocyte ploidy, and when
DNA synthesis is impaired, megakaryocyte
ploidy is abnormally low (Bessman 1984), with a
consequent low MPV. Note that the megakaryocyte and platelet defect is fully corrected by
therapy. In contrast, patients with aplastic anemia who have recovered normal platelt counts
have a persistent low MPV. In the rare hereditary Wiskott-Aldrich syndrome, thrombocytopenia
is accompanied by small and hypofunctional
platelets (Lum et al. 1980).

When bone marrow infiltration by fibrosis or
neoplastic cells does not lower the platelet
count, MPV is normal. When infiltration so
compromises normal hematopoiesis that the
platelet count is low, then the MPV also usually
is inappropriately low.

Just as asplenia is accompanied by thrombocytosis and increased MPV, hypersplenism is
accompanied by thrombocytopenia and low MPV
(Karpatkin and Freedman 1978), further suggest-

ing that the spleen preferentially culls the largest platelets.

Our experience is that 28 subjects with thrombocytopenia and appropriately increased MPV always had normal-to-increased megakaryocytes in their bone marrow, whereas 59 subjects with inappropriately low MPV (for the platelet count) had reduced (46 patients) or normal (13) megakaryocytes in hypoplastic or infiltrated bone marrow. If others' experience is similar, evaluation of peripheral-blood MPV may replace bone marrow examination of megakaryocytes in selected cases.

Alcoholics may have mild or severe thrombocytopenia. Just as there are multiple causes of the abnormal red cell values seen in such patients, the causes of the platelet abnormality include direct marrow toxicity, peripheral platelet destruction, folate deficiency, and hypersplenism (Sahud 1972). Depending on the cause, MPV may be appropriately high for the reduced platelet count or may not.

3.8 Sequential Studies of Platelet Size during a Disease Course

3.8.1 *Immune Thrombocytopenia*

As described in section 3.5, ITP is accompanied by increased MPV inversely but nonlinearly related to platelet count. This relation seems to be an extension of the same relation among normal subjects. The sequential data in individuals during a changing course of ITP also illustrate the same relation. Figure 3.11 shows that, at the nadir of thrombocytopenia, MPV is at a maximum. As platelet count rises during remission of ITP, MPV falls. When the platelet count reaches a normal value, MPV likewise is the same as in normal subjects. This illustrates two points. First, increased MPV is associated not with all immune platelet destruction, but only with immune destruction accompanied by thrombocytopenia—

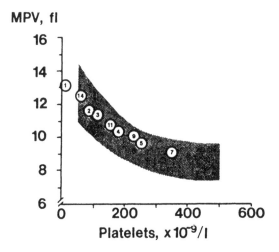

MPV, fl

FIGURE 3.14
*Immune thrombocyto-
penic purpura. The
circled numbers show the
sequential days after
prednisone was given.
During recovery, as platelet count rose, MPV fell,
until a normal platelet
count and MPV were
reached. After prednisone
was stopped, platelet
count fell and MPV rose,
with values matching
those during recovery.
Source for figures 3.14–
3.16: adapted from Bess-
man and Gardner 1983.*

that is, where the bone marrow cannot fully
compensate for the platelet destruction. When
the increased peripheral platelet destruction is
sufficiently moderate to allow the marrow to
compensate with a normal platelet count, MPV is
entirely normal. As noted earlier, this is an
analog of the association of macrocytosis and
anemia in immune hemolytic disorders (section
2.6.2.).

Second, the progressive course in figure 3.14
shows that platelet size is not chiefly determined
by platelet age. During the rapid rise in platelet
count, each day the majority of platelets are
newly formed, yet each day the MPV falls (Levin
and Bessman 1983; Bessman and Gardner
1983). Newly formed platelets, therefore, must
occur in various sizes, depending on megakaryocyte stimulation. This, too, parallels the relation between reticulocytes and erythroid
stimulation.

If thrombocytopenia is severe enough, the few
genuine platelets may be obscured by low-level
background noise as well as by the erythrocyte
and platelet fragments that accompany severe
ITP (Shulman et al. 1982; Zucker-Franklin and
Karpatkin 1977). MPV will be unreliable by the

MPV, fl

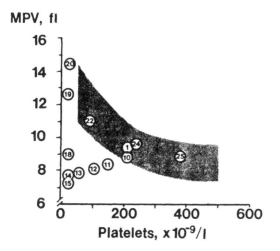

Platelets, x 10⁻⁹/l

FIGURE 3.15

Cytotoxic chemotherapy. The circled numbers show the days after anti-leukemic chemotherapy. On days 1–10, both platelet count and MPV are normal. On day 11, platelet count has fallen slightly but still is in the normal range; MPV also has fallen, so that it is abnormally small for the platelet count. By day 15 a minimum of platelet count and MPV is reached. The first recovery is of MPV (days 18 and 19), then platelet count rises (day 20). As platelet count rises further (days 22–25), MPV falls in the same manner as in the reference pattern from normals.

instrument's calculation. MPV will become determinable and high as the first sign of recovery of platelet count, indicating that the low platelet count now reflects platelets rather than primarily noise (Levin and Bessman 1983). Then, as platelet count rises, MPV falls as described.

3.8.2 *Cytotoxic Chemotherapy*

When the bone marrow is suppressed, MPV does not rise appropriately as platelet count falls. Therefore, as shown in figure 3.15, as the platelet count falls after marrow supression by cytotoxic chemotherapy, MPV is progressively more abnormally low. The nadir of platelet count also is the point of the maximum difference in MPV between hypoproductive thrombocytopenia (shown here) and hyperdestructive thrombocytopenia (fig. 3.14). During recovery, megakaryocytes begin to increase their DNA content. The higher-DNA megakaryocytes make larger platelets, which cause a rise in MPV. This is generally the first sign of marrow recovery: MPV rises while platelet count is still low. One to two days later, platelet count begins to rise, and MPV then falls as platelet count continues to rise to normal.

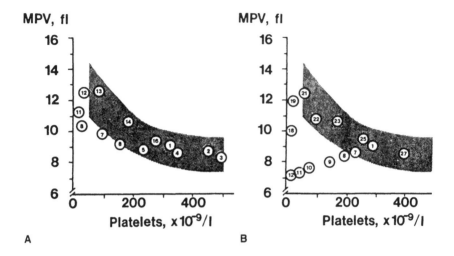

3.8.3 *Sepsis*

Sepsis often is accompanied by thrombocytopenia. Both increased destruction and
marrow suppression may be responsible. Serial
examinations of MPV and platelet count will
show that the patterns often are intermediate,
suggesting a multifactorial cause of thrombocytopenia (fig. 3.16) (Bessman and Gardner
1983). An important use of these data in septic
patients is in anticipating recovery: if the bone
marrow is suppressed (low platelet count, low
MPV), recovery can be expected soon after, but
not until, MPV rises. A fall in MPV suggests that
the bone marrow has ceased compensatory increases in megakaryocytopoiesis. In our surgical
intensive care unit, 50 percent of such patients
recovered, and about 50 percent died. They did
not die of hemorrhage. In contrast, all patients
survived whose MPV did not fall during the development of thrombocytopenia. This distinction
suggests that lack of marrow compensation to
produce increased MPV during thrombocytopenia predicts a particularly compromised
individual. It is the compromised state, not the
thrombocytopenia, that is so often fatal.

MPV, fl

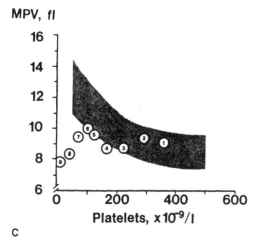

C

FIGURE 3.16
Septic thrombocytopenia. Depending on whether the thrombocytopenia is caused by purely increased platelet destruction (a) or purely marrow suppression (b), the MPV will change as in ITP or as in cytotoxic chemotherapy. Often there is an intermediate pattern to suggest some degree of both causes. If MPV is low during the nadir of platelet count, it will rise before platelet count; (c) A patient with lymphoma and pneumococcal pneumonia. As platelet count fell, MPV rose slightly and remained in the nomogram, suggesting marrow compensation (days 1–6). On days 7 and 8, MPV fell, diverging from the nomogram, although platelet count still was near-normal. This signaled a loss of marrow compensation; both MPV and platelet count fell, and the patient did not recover.

Hemorrhage occurs more often in subjects with low rather than high MPV (Eldor, Avitzour, and Or 1982). Large platelets may be hemostatically more active (Karpatkin 1978), but in addition, subjects with low MPV often have prolonged thrombocytopenia due to malignancy or aplasia. Patients with septic thrombocytopenia did not have abnormal bleeding, regardless of MPV: the brief spell of thrombocytopenia ended in either recovery or death. Subjects with prolonged extreme thrombocytopenia may have an incremental risk of bleeding over time. In these cases it is especially important to examine the peripheral blood smear and the platelet distribution histogram. In subjects with platelets $<10 \times 10^9/l$, if platelets are seen and the histogram is normal shaped, bleeding is far less likely than if no platelets are seen and the histogram shows the artifacts discussed in the next section (our experience).

3.9 Artifacts

As noted for red cells, these are true biologic abnormalities that can be identified by abnormal automated blood counts. When the platelet count is normal, nonplatelet particles rarely are numer-

A

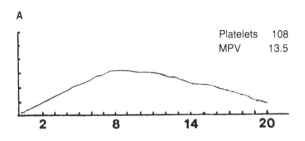

Platelets   108
MPV   13.5

B

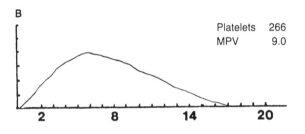

Platelets   266
MPV   9.0

FIGURE 3.17

Platelet clumping in EDTA. Although the automated blood count (a) showed a reduced platelet count, a high MPV, and an irregular platelet volume histogram, the peripheral blood smear showed abundant clumped platelets. (b) Citrate-anticoagulated blood yields a normal platelet count, although the MPV is about 20 percent less in citrate than in the usual EDTA anticoagulant.

ous enough to affect the platelet count or MPV. The more severe the thrombocytopenia, the more likely these artifacts will affect the results.

3.9.1 *Platelet Clumping*

Occasional patients' platelets clump in EDTA. This causes the automated platelet count to fall proportional to the clumping (Shreiner and Bell 1973). The volume of clumped platelets is far less than the sum of volume of the individual platelets that have become attached. This is because of the changed "shape factor," which is more important for platelets than for red cells. Because only particles 2–20 fl are measured as platelets, those clumps measured at >20 fl will not be counted even as one platelet. The platelet volume histogram may be modestly changed from log-normal; however, because the clumps are numerically relatively few, this is not a reliable indicator. Rather, when visual review of the blood smear shows many more platelets than the automated count, clumping may be suspected (fig. 3.17). The definitive demonstration is

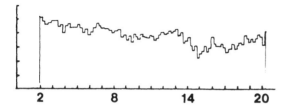

FIGURE 3.18
The effect of nonplatelet fragments. Red cell fragments merge with platelets, increasing both the platelet count and the MPV. In this case the instrument did not provide a value for platelet count or MPV; the phase-microscopy platelet count was 17 × 10⁹/l.

measurement of citrate-anticoagulated blood. The platelets will not clump, and an accurate automated count will be obtained. Note, however, that the EDTA-induced platelet shape change does not occur with citrate anti-coagulation. Therefore, the MPV in citrate-anticoagulated blood will be approximately 20 percent below the MPV of the nonclumped platelets in EDTA. This example stresses the importance of correlating abnormal automated values with the peripheral blood smear.

3.9.2 Red Cell Fragments

As noted previously, red cell fragments >36 fl will be counted as red cells and artifactually lower the MCV. In contrast, red cell fragments <20 fl will be counted as platelets (Zucker-Franklin and Karpatkin 1977). Platelet count will be spuriously elevated; MPV will be altered to reflect the size of the fragment (Bessman, Williams, and Gilmer 1981; Akwari, Ross, and Stass 1982; Gilmer, Williams, and Bessman 1982; Cornbleet and Kessinger 1985). The platelet volume histogram will be manifestly different from log-normal (fig. 3.18), providing a clue to detection of this artifact. Slow, brief centrifugation of the whole blood will sediment the red cell fragments to the red cell layer, leaving fragment-free platelet-rich plasma. Platelet counting and sizing from the platelet-rich plasma will yield accurate data about the actual platelets (Bessman, Williams, and Gilmer 1981). Any of the disorders causing red cell fragmentation listed in section

TABLE 3.4 Duplicate Error in Platelet Counts

Nominal Count (× 10⁹/l)	Duplicate Error (%)
< 10	100
10–20	50
20–40	33
40–80	20
80–160	15
160–320	10
>320	5

Note: These figures are for automated counts; duplicate error is at least 50 percent greater for visual techniques.

2.7.1 may cause this artifact. Likewise, red cells with an extremely low MCV (<65 fl) may be distributed to include a few intact red cells <20 fl, producing the same effect.

3.9.3 Blast Fragments

A similar artifact will be caused by fragments of leukemic blasts, in either acute or chronic leukemia (Bessman, Williams, and Gilmer 1981). Fragments of reactive neutrophils also rarely may mimic platelets (Hanker and Giammara 1983).

3.9.4 Extreme Thrombocytopenia

The duplicate error of the automated platelet count is approximately as shown in table 3.4. The duplicate error on visual phase counts is greater. Therefore, platelet counts <10 × 10⁹/l cannot be distinguished from each other. When platelet count is sufficiently low, the signal-to-noise ratio may be treacherously high (Cornbleet and Kessinger 1985). In these cases the platelet volume distribution histogram is of particular value. If the histogram is log-normally shaped as in normal subjects, then the platelet count and MPV are likely to reflect blood platelets reliably. In contrast, if the distribution histogram is not log-normal, the platelet count and MPV are likely

A

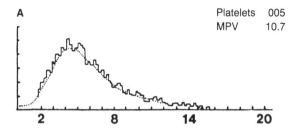

| Platelets | 005 |
| MPV | 10.7 |

B

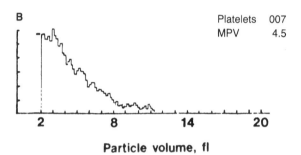

| Platelets | 007 |
| MPV | 4.5 |

Particle volume, fl

FIGURE 3.19

Extreme thrombocyto-penia. (a) The platelet histogram is log-normal, in-dicating that platelets are being counted despite the low platelet count. (b) The platelet histogram is inde-terminate, indicating that platelets are not being counted reliably.

to represent only background noise (fig. 3.19). Importantly, such results are equally unreliable whether the thrombocytopenia is associated with large or small platelets. Thus, if the platelet count is $<10 \times 10^9/l$, MPV may be unreliable to distinguish the cause. Such unreliable results can be identified by the non-log-normal histogram.

If the histogram is abnormal enough, some in-struments may not report any platelet values.

4
White Cells

4.1 Introduction

Leukocytes are divided into discrete morphologic subsets: commonly, segmented neutrophils, bands, metamyelocytes, promyelocytes, blasts, basophils, eosinophils, lymphocytes, monocytes, and variant lymphocytes. In the visual differential, their relative proportion is found among 100 or 200 cells. However, two technical problems limit the value of visual differentials. First, the duplicate error in counting the cell types is quite large: up to 100 percent for cells <10 percent of the total, and >25 percent for even the most common types, neutrophils or lymphocytes (Rumke 1975; Koepke 1978). Second, the intra-observer variation is equally high in distinguishing "bands" from mature neutrophils and monocytes, or atypical lymphocytes from lymphocytes. Substantial variations in the differential, especially in the band count, may be caused more by technique than biology (Koepke 1985). Because visual differentials are time intensive, recognition of these difficulties has led to various strategies to limit their use (Rock and Grogan 1983; Rich, Crowson, and Connelly 1983; Koepke 1985). Generally these strategies stipulate limits of "normality" within which the differential is unlikely to provide useful information if performed. Also, users increasingly question the threshold at which results are abnormal enough to warrant further investigation.

Certainly even one blast on the peripheral smear is too many, and if this is a new finding, further investigation always is appropriate. However, what is the percentage above which eosinophilia and monocytosis is abnormal? Absolute monocyte or eosinophil counts only partially address this issue, because the absolute counts are the product of total leukocyte count times the monocyte or eosinophil percentage. Therefore, the absolute count is no more reliable than the reliability of the monocyte or eosinophil percentage. The clinician must be uncertain in many cases whether a monocyte or eosinophil value in the broad ambiguous zone should be evaluated further or not (Koepke 1978).

Into this uncertainty has been introduced automated analysis of white cells. There are three general methods, described below, each of which eliminates the two technical difficulties of the visual differential. All measure at least several hundred white cells, making statistical variation far less important. Each also relies on stipulated, programmed criteria for cell identification, eliminating inter- or intraobserver variation. Each of these techniques has substituted new criteria for the pattern recognition of Wright-Giemsa cytochemistry, to some degree subjective and personal, with which the technologist and clinician are familiar. Nuclear-cytoplasmic ratio, cell area and shape, nuclear shape, granule content, and color all play a part in the "neuro-optical system" of slide analysis.

Image analysis is the automated technology that is based on the most familiar criteria, because the variables are essentially the same as for light microscopy. The difference is that the criteria are applied more regularly with automation. In contrast, flow-impedance and flow-cytochemistry leukocyte analysis are based on completely new criteria, as described in individual sections below. The user of these technologies should appreciate that the nonmorphological criteria have been adjusted to match, *on average,* the results obtained by morphology. In individual patients, there is only an assumption that the data will match, unless a microscopic differential is done each time. On the other hand, with new criteria for classification, abnormalities indetectable by light microscopy will appear. These abnormalities are only now being evaluated.

To date, the primary thrust of the automated differential has been to allow a screening procedure to reduce the number of time- and labor-intensive visual differentials. For this purpose a high correlation coefficient between manual and automated differentials may be reassuring (Hansen and Stahl 1984). However, the automated differential gives incomplete information about the less common normal, or about abnormal cells. No automated instrument at present reliably identifies cell types less common than 1 percent of the total. Therefore, the visual white cell differential cannot always be replaced by this automated procedure (Cox et al. 1985; Savage 1985). Two general approaches are being considered. One approach is to develop a set of screening criteria based on the complete blood count and, only when certain abnormalities are found, then to add the visual differential as a "special test" (B. S. Bull, personal communication; Pierre 1985, with discussion). The other approach is routinely to perform a visual examination of the first blood specimen from a given patient, but then to repeat the visual differential only for some stipulated criteria (Nelson et al. 1985; Dutcher 1985; Mayer 1985). Development of these criteria will be affected by the proportion of normal and abnormal samples that form the laboratory's mix, and the type of abnormalities seen. The general-practice office, pediatric intensive care unit, and employee health clinic may have different needs. Furthermore, some laboratories may report only numerical values and not the histograms or scattergrams. To date, little interpretation has been made of the automated white cell differentials except for precision, accuracy, and quality control.

Our current policy has been developed for blood specimens of inpatients at a tertiary hospital and for outpatients of the hematology and oncology clinics. We recognize that our workload includes more hematologic abnormalities than those of most laboratories:

1. The first specimen has both an automated blood count and differential, and visual review of morphology and formal 100-cell leukocyte differential. All results are reported. This assures detection of the following abnormalities that may not be detected by any automated instrument:

Granulocytes: rare abnormal cells (blasts, promyelocytes, myelocytes, basophils, nucleated red cells, hairy cells, Sézary cells). If these are more than 3 percent of the total, often they will be "flagged" (see below) in Coulter systems. Less common normal cells in abnormal percentage (eosinophils, monocytes, variant lymphocytes). If more than 5 percent, often these will be "flagged" (see below). Morphologic abnormalities (Pelger-Huet, toxic granulation, hypersegmentation)

Erythrocytes: sickled cells, burrs, targets, spheres; rouleaux; basophilic stippling; Howell-Jolly bodies; polychromasia; fragments, teardrop cells

Platelets: bizarre morphology; clumping

Each of these except for promyelocytes has been seen in subjects having automated blood counts without other abnormal values. However, in our experience, such undetected abnormalities occur in less than one-quarter of 1 percent of normal blood counts.

2. Subsequent specimens have only the automated blood count and differential unless:
   a. there is a twofold increase or decrease from the last WBC count;
   b. any histogram changes enough for new flagging signals;
   c. there is an identified need for visual examination (e.g., a leukemic patient in possible relapse versus remission);
   d. the responsible physician requests visual examination; for this, no reason is needed.

Note that by these rules even subjects with extremely low counts may not require serial visual examination as long as the underlying abnormality is known and the automated data do not change. This has reduced the need for visual differentials by 75 percent. In the 1,000 visual differentials done before this policy that would have been omitted with this policy, no new abnormality would have been missed by omitting the visual differential.

This or similar approaches will be facilitated by a computer-based decision system in larger laboratories (Dutcher 1985).

Far less has been done to use the automated information to define new diseases. Because the automated differential is based on new criteria, it is to be expected that abnormalities will be found that are unrelated to detectable light-microscopic abnormalities. These studies are largely still in the future. This section is meant only to explain the present use of automated differentials and the interpretation of common, well-understood and well-characterized white cell disorders.

The differential diagnosis of an increase or decrease in each particular leukocyte subset (e.g., lymphopenia, eosinophilia) is long, and well described in standard texts (Stein 1983; Williams 1983; Wintrobe 1981).

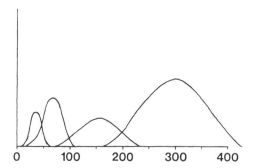

e of the
Coulter three-part white
cell differential. The volume scale is in femtoli-
ters. Nucleated red cells
register at 40–60; lymphocytes at 50–99; "mono-
nuclear" cells at 100–160;
and neutrophils at
160–400. Leukemic
blasts, atypical lympho-
cytes, eosinophils, Sézary
cells, hairy cells, plasma
cells, and basophils also
are found in the 90–180 fl
range (our experience;
Pierre 1984; Ward 1985).

4.2   Flow Measurements: Nuclear Volume

The principle of the Coulter flow differential is
that the nuclei of the several cell types have distinctly different sizes. After incubation of the
leukocytes in a liquid of particular tonicity, the
cytoplasm is nominally leached out and the cell
membrane collapsed about the nucleus (England, Chetty, and DeSilva 1982). The present
generation of counters (Coulter S-Plus IV, V, and
VI) are based on a diluent that produces four relatively distinct nuclear size peaks: nucleated red
cells; lymphocytes; granulocytes; and other cells.
The composite curve is shown schematically in
figure 4.1. In contrast to red cells and platelets,
the scale on the white cell volume distribution
histogram does not correspond even to a nominal whole-cell volume, but instead to a nominal
nuclear volume. The volume scale is similar for
white cell nuclei and for intact erythrocytes. As is
the case for the other cell types, the information
from the numbers is complemented by examination of the histogram by the clinician and/or the
laboratory. The curves and "flags" shown below
are for the Coulter instrument. Other instruments
(e.g., the Toa Sysmex E-5000 and Sequoia-
Turner Cell Dyn-2000) offer three-part nuclear-
volume leukocyte differentials that are under
investigation (Bessman, unpublished data; R. V.
Pierre, personal communication).

4.2.1 *Normal Values*

The distribution of leukocytes in normal subjects varies individually and also from day to day. With visual differentials, it is probable that this is in part because of technical error, but there also is biologic variation. The degree of variation of an automated differential over time in normal subjects is not yet well documented. It is likely that the variation will be less and reflect more exclusively biologic variation than do the values obtained with serial visual differentials. Normal values in adults, based on visual differentials, are approximately:

	Percentage	Absolute, $\times 10^9$/l
neutrophils	45–80	1.8–8.0
bands	0–5	0–0.5
lymphocytes	15–45	1.2–4.2
monocytes	0–10	0–1.0
eosinophils	0–5	0–0.5
basophils	0–3	0–0.3

Nucleated red cells, blasts, or myelocytes seen on the peripheral smear are prima facie evidence of an abnormality.

A normal distribution of leukocyte nuclear size shows a clear peak of lymphocytes, a clear peak of granulocytes, and a variable lower plateau between these two peaks that corresponds to "mononuclear cells." In the Coulter instrument, granulocytes generally appear in the "granulocyte" region >200 fl, but occasionally will appear below 200 fl and even in the "mononuclear" area. No specific disorder is associated with such cases (fig. 4.2). If the granulocyte or lymphocyte peak is obscured, the distribution will be "flagged" in one or more leukocyte types. The most abnormal histograms will have no numbers reported. Listed below are abnormalities that in one or more instances have caused this flagging. However, all subjects with these

A

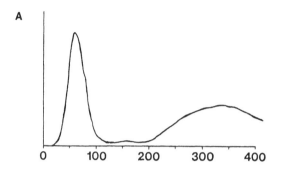

B

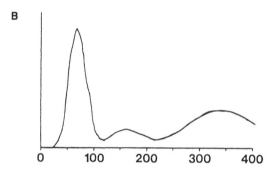

C

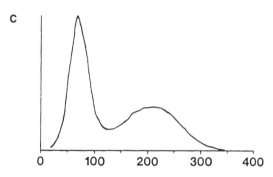

FIGURE 4.2
Different appearances of "normal" neutrophils. In each case the manual differential showed 45 percent lymphocytes, 50 percent neutrophils, and 5 percent monocytes. (a) Neutrophils all are within a single peak (mean 340 fl). The automated differential showed 43 percent lymphocytes, 8 percent mononuclears and 48 percent granulocytes. (b) Neutrophils are partially in the granulocyte area, partially in the mononuclear area. The automated differential was 47 percent lymphocytes, 14 percent mononuclears, and 39 percent granulocytes. (c) Neutrophils are substantially within the mononuclear area. The automated differential was 46 percent lymphocytes, 21 percent mononuclears, and 33 percent granulocytes.

abnormalities will not be flagged, nor will all flagged differentials be due to one of these disorders.

R1 (left of lymphocyte peak): malaria, parasites, cryoglobulins, platelets, nucleated red cells, sickled cells.

R2 (right side of lymphocyte peak): basophils, blasts, variant lymphocytes, plasma cells, hairy cells, Sézary cells.

R3 (left side of granulocyte peak): abnormally migrating granulocytes, eosinophils, myelocytes.

R4 (right side of granulocyte peak): unknown.

The correlation between 5,000 visually determined and 5,000 Coulter S-Plus IV impedance leukocyte percentages in our hospital, was:

Neutrophils   r = 0.99
Monocytes   r = 0.48 (to "mononuclear" cells)
Lymphocytes r = 0.99

Similar correlations have been reported by several laboratories (Savage 1985; Pierre 1985; Nelson et al. 1985).

Because of the variability in normal differentials, no single distribution histogram can be used as a template against which to judge normal and abnormal results. Blacks have leukocyte counts about 20 percent lower than whites (table 2.1).

4.2.2 *Granulocytosis and Lymphopenia*

In infection or inflammation, granulocytes may be absolutely increased, or relatively increased because of lymphocytopenia. In either case the lymphocyte peak is relatively reduced, and the granulocyte peak is increased (fig. 4.3). Distinction between these two types of disorder depends on the absolute count of the different cell types.

4.2.3 *Lymphocytosis and Granulocytopenia*

Lymphocytes may be absolutely increased, as in, for example, chronic lymphocytic leukemia (CLL), or may be relatively increased by absolute granulocytopenia (fig. 4.4) (see section 4.2). Absolute leukocyte counts will distinguish between these two causes. CLL lymphocytes generally show the same nuclear volume as do

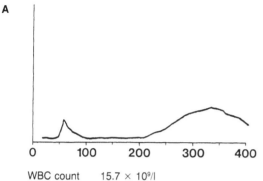

A

WBC count   15.7 × 10⁹/l
Differential: Automated Visual
    Granulocytes   87   79   Neutrophils
                                8   Bands
                                2   Eosinophils
    Mononuclear   4   3   Monocytes
    Lymphocytes   9   8   Lymphocytes

B

WBC count   5.3 × 10⁹/l
Differential: Automated Visual
    Granulocytes   86   88   Neutrophils
                                0   Bands
                                1   Eosinophils
    Mononuclear   6   4   Monocytes
    Lymphocytes   8   7   Lymphocytes

FIGURE 4.3
Granulocytosis. (a) Neu-trophilia. The neutrophil percentage is increased, with an increased granu-locyte peak. (b) Lympho-penia. The pattern is the same as above, in this case due to reduced lymphocytes.

normal lymphocytes (fig. 4.4a). Occasionally, especially during the late stages, poorly differ-entiated CLL lymphocytes will have larger-than-normal nuclei both on peripheral smear and on distribution histogram.

A

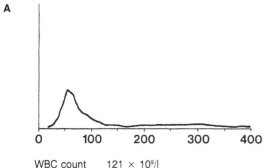

WBC count	121 × 10⁹/l		
Differential:	Automated	Visual	
Granulocytes	1	2	Neutrophils
		0	Bands
		0	Eosinophils
Mononuclear	2	1	Monocytes
Lymphocytes	97	97	Lymphocytes

B

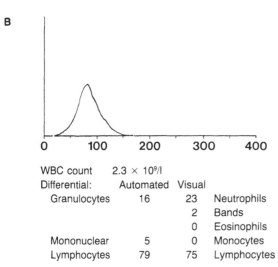

WBC count	2.3 × 10⁹/l		
Differential:	Automated	Visual	
Granulocytes	16	23	Neutrophils
		2	Bands
		0	Eosinophils
Mononuclear	5	0	Monocytes
Lymphocytes	79	75	Lymphocytes

FIGURE 4.4
Lymphocytosis. (a) Chronic lymphocytic leukemia (CLL). Nearly all cells appear between 50 and 100 fl. The lymphocytes are morphologically normal. (b) Neutropenia. The histogram is the same as above. However, the total leukocyte count is low instead of high, and there is absolute neutropenia.

4.2.4 *Eosinophilia*

Eosinophils appear in an intermediate position overlapping the "mononuclear" and granulocyte areas of the white cell histogram, despite the morphologic difference between them and either of the other cell types. The differential is quite

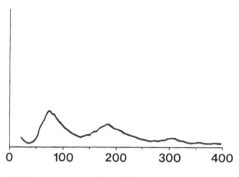

WBC count	11.6 × 10⁹/l		
Differential:	Automated	Visual	
Granulocytes	45	41	Neutrophils
		1	Bands
		30	Eosinophils
Mononuclear	27	3	Monocytes
Lymphocytes	28	25	Lymphocytes

FIGURE 4.5

Eosinophilia. The visually determined 30 percent eosinophils correlates well with the automated 27 percent mononuclear cells. Here, as in the next section, the increased mononuclear percentage should prompt visual examination to determine which cell type is being counted, as "mononuclear" in the automated differential.

long for diagnosis of eosinophilia (Stein 1983). It remains to be determined, when increased precision is available with automated differentials, whether the same disorders will continue to be associated with eosinophilia (fig. 4.5). It should be emphasized that the intermediate apparent size of the eosinophil nucleus is similar to the size of monocytes, some abnormal cells, and occasionally granulocytes. Therefore, the presence of increased "mononuclear" cells is not a specific indication of eosinophilia. However, when eosinophilia exceeds 10 percent, there will reliably be an increase in "mononuclear" cells and/or a "flag" in the Coulter differential. Marked eosinophilia may be detectable by other types of automated differentials (fig. 4.12b).

4.2.5 *Monocytosis*

Monocytes also appear in the "mononuclear" area of the white cell histogram. The differential diagnosis of monocytosis again is quite lengthy, though monocytosis is found only occasionally in

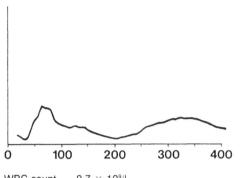

WBC count   9.7 × 10⁹/l

Differential:	Automated	Visual	
Granulocytes	50	55	Neutrophils
		2	Bands
		1	Eosinophils
Mononuclear	21	18	Monocytes
Lymphocytes	29	24	Lymphocytes

FIGURE 4.6

Monocytosis. The percentage of monocytes in the visual differential was 18 percent, correlating well with the automated percentage of mononuclear cells, 21 percent. Visual examination distinguishes this from a similar automated differential caused by eosinophilia (fig. 4.5) or by atypically migrating granulocytes (fig. 4.2).

most such disorders. Monocytes are less clearly distinguishable from other leukocytes than are eosinophils by light microscopy. Mononuclear percentages are more reproducible in automated techniques than are monocyte percentages in visual techniques (Koepke 1978; Koepke 1985). However, as noted in section 4.2.4, in the automated differential monocytes and eosinophils (as well as other rarer cells described elsewhere in the chapter) will be confused. Therefore, the correlation between the Coulter mononuclear percentage and the manual monocyte percentage is only about $r = 0.50$. Other instruments do not appear to have a higher correlation. Whether an increased automated "mononuclear" percentage is caused by monocytes, eosinophils, or other cells must be determined by a visual differential. However, monocytosis >10 percent by visual microscopy registers as monocytosis >10 percent by the Coulter differential (63 of 65 cases) (fig. 4.6). The variability of the manual percentage of monocytes may partially account for

A

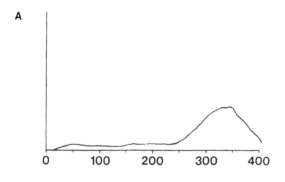

B

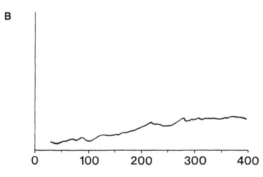

FIGURE 4.7
Chronic myelogenous leukemia. (a) Early phase. The white cell count is 23 × 10⁹/l. The visual differential is: granulocytes 57 percent, bands 29 percent, myelocytes 8 percent, monocytes 1 percent, eosinophils 2 percent, basophils 1 percent, lymphocytes 2 percent. The automated differential does not suggest any immature cells. (b) Late phase. The white cell count is 98 × 10⁹/l. The visual differential is: granulocytes 56 percent, bands 18 percent, myelocytes 13 percent, promyelocytes 3 percent, blasts 2 percent, monocytes 1 percent, eosinophils 2 percent, basophils 3 percent, lymphocytes 2 percent. The automated histogram shows a single, broad distribution. Although the differential is only moderately different from that in panel a, the histogram is markedly more abnormal. The morphologic basis for this difference is not yet clear.

the poor correlation of slight monocytosis with individual disorders.

4.2.6 Chronic Myelogenous Leukemia and Myelofibrosis/Myelodysplasia

In two diseases, chronic myelogenous leukemia and myelofibrosis, there is a marked shift from mature to immature neutrophils in the peripheral blood. There is an increased proportion of myelocytes, promyelocytes, nucleated red cells, and sometimes blasts. The histogram of white cell nuclear volume often shows a single, broadly distributed population of cells with or without a separate lymphocyte population (fig. 4.7). The more advanced the myeloproliferative disorder, the more bizarre the distribution: the markedly abnormal pattern shown in figure 4.7b would not

A

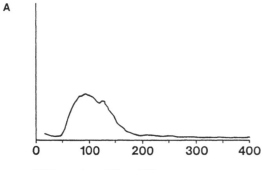

WBC count	5.9 × 10⁹/l		
Differential:	Automated	Visual	
Granulocytes	Not	27	Neutrophils
	Reported	5	Bands
	due to	0	Eosinophils
Mononuclear	abnormal	3	Monocytes
Lymphocytes	histogram	45	Lymphocytes
		20	Blasts

B

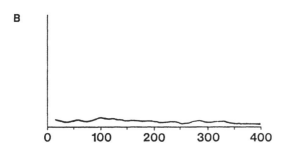

WBC count	0.3 × 10⁹/l		
Differential:	Automated	Visual	(Based on 10 cells)
Granulocytes	Not	50	Neutrophils
	Reported	0	Bands
	due to	0	Eosinophils
Mononuclear	abnormal	30	Monocytes
Lymphocytes	histogram	20	Lymphocytes

C

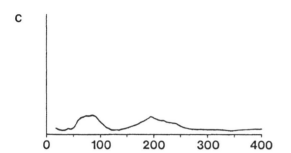

WBC count   0.6 × 10⁹/l

Differential:	Automated	Visual	(Based on 50 cells)
Granulocytes	34	28	Neutrophils
		10	Bands
		6	Eosinophils
Mononuclear	15	8	Monocytes
Lymphocytes	51	48	Lymphocytes

D

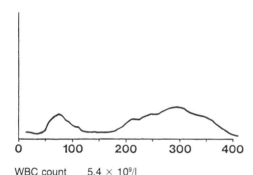

WBC count   5.4 × 10⁹/l

Differential:	Automated	Visual	
Granulocytes	59	61	Neutrophils
		0	Bands
		1	Eosinophils
Mononuclear	7	5	Monocytes
Lymphocytes	44	43	Lymphocytes

FIGURE 4.8
Serial white cell distributions during bone marrow suppression by cytotoxic chemotherapy, and subsequent recovery. The visual differential counts are shown. (a) Pretherapy. There is only one peak of cells. The volume is slightly larger than lymphocytes, and these are blast cells, as was found in the peripheral smear. Since this peak did not conform to the automated criteria, there was no automated differential reported. (b) At the nadir of white count. Essentially no leukocytes are present, and neither the automated nor the visual differential is accurate. (c) Early recovery. Lymphocytes, mononuclear cells, and a few granulocytes appear. Although the leukocyte count still is very low, the automated differential correlated well with the visual differential. (d) Full recovery. Both the number and the type of leukocytes are normal. Note that the lymphocyte peak differs from that of the blasts. Again the automated and visual differentials correlated well.

be likely in a patient with early chronic myelogenous leukemia who was untreated, and had
only a moderate elevation of leukocytes.

4.2.7 *Acute Leukemia*

Drug therapy of acute leukemia is intended to
produce bone marrow suppression of limited
duration and severity. During this suppression,
granulocyte counts fall (fig. 4.8a,b). During subsequent recovery the white cell count rises. During the first days of increasing white count after
marrow recovery there may be an increased percentage of monocytes (fig. 4.8c), and then a return to mature granulocytes (fig. 4.8d).

The visual differential count is particularly difficult when the total white cell count is low: the
differential may be of fewer cells, or the increased search for white cells may increase
observer error or bias. The same is true of the
volume histogram, in that the fewer the cells
counted, the less well characterized are the separate populations (fig. 4.8b,c). Only if the peaks
are clearly identifiable can the automated differential be relied upon (fig. 4.8d).

Figure 4.8a shows that blast cells appear at a
slightly different peak than do lymphocytes. This
is apparent when many blasts are in the peripheral blood. However, if <10 percent blasts are
present, no abnormal peak will be seen. Thus,
an abnormal peak alerts the reader to a probable abnormal blood smear. A normal histogram
does not relieve the reader of the need to review
the blood smear for occasional blasts, should
that be indicated.

4.2.8 *Nucleated Red Cells*

Most nucleated red cells in the peripheral blood
are the most mature form, with pyknotic nuclei
that are smaller than those of lymphocytes. Their
mean volume is approximately 55 fl on this
scale, in contrast to 70 fl for lymphocytes. The
appearance of the histogram depends on the

A

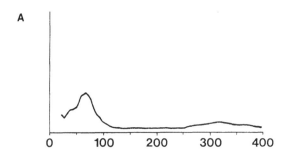

B

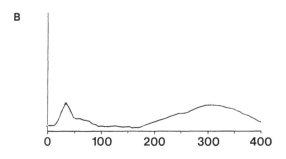

FIGURE 4.9
Nucleated red cells. (a) 5 percent nucleated red cells. There is a bulge at the left of the lymphocyte peak. This bulge is characteristic of nucleated red cells when they are fewer than the lymphocytes. (b) 32 percent nucleated red cells. The lymphocytes are few, and so a relatively pure nucleated red cell peak is seen, at a smaller mean value than lymphocytes.

relative number of nucleated red cells and lymphocytes. If lymphocytes are absent, even 3 nucleated red cells per 100 white cells will produce a distinct peak (fig. 4.9a). If lymphocytes are more numerous, the peak of nucleated red cells will fuse with that of the lymphocytes (fig. 4.9b), but still as few as 8 percent will cause a characteristic alteration in the histogram. Either pattern is highly suggestive of nucleated red cells. The most common causes are erythroid hyperplasia associated with asplenia (e.g., hemoglobin SS), myelophthisis, or immune hemolytic anemia.

4.2.9 *Other Cells*

Myelocytes, basophils, plasma cells, and other rare cells very uncommonly appear in the peripheral blood in a number large enough (>10 percent of total) to appear as a peak in these histograms. Further experience is needed in these rare cases. When such cells are less

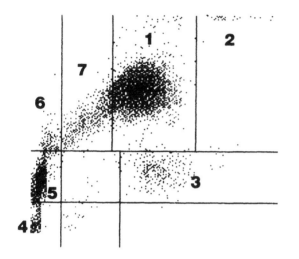

FIGURE 4.10
Cytochemical differential. Light scatter is measured on the vertical axis and absorption (myeloperoxi- dase content) on the horizontal axis. (1) neutro- phils, (2) high peroxidase activity, (3) eosinophils, (4) platelets, RBC debris, noise, (5) lymphocytes, (6) large unstained cells (LUC), and (7) mono- cytes, basophils. Source: Copyright 1982 Technicon Instruments Corporation, Tarrytown, New York.

common, the distribution histogram may be "flagged," or they may be found only by visual inspection of the blood smear.

Band-form neutrophils are not identified as different from polymorphonuclear neutrophils by any of the flow-cytometry instruments. The value of routine band percentages remains contro- versial (Nelson et al. 1985). The "high- peroxidase" cells in the Technicon cytochemical differential (see fig. 4.10 and section 4.3) may correlate with toxic granulation of neutrophils.

4.3 Flow Measurements: Enzyme Content

The principle of the Technicon flow differential (e.g., hemalog D, H6000/601C, or H1) is that different cell types have different size (light scatter) and different content of the enzyme myeloperoxidase. The cells are incubated in a reagent to produce a color reaction proportional to single cell enzyme content. A scattergram then is developed of all cells that are measured in a stipulated time (e.g., three seconds), with size on the vertical axis and myeloperoxidase content on the horizontal. A normal distribution is

A
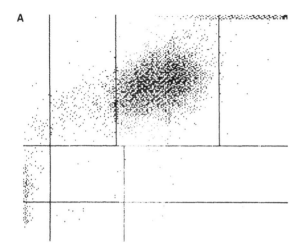

B
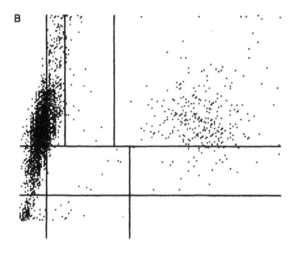

FIGURE 4.11
Cytochemical differential. (a) Neutrophilia. (b) Blast transformation in chronic myeloid leukemia (note the preponderance of cells in the large un- stained cell area). Source: Copyright 1983 Technicon Instruments Corporation, Tarrytown, New York.

shown in figure 4.10, and abnormal scattergrams are shown in figures 4.11 and 4.12. This tech- nology shows five classes of leukocytes: neu- trophils, lymphocytes, monocytes, eosinophils, and "large unstained cells," which often cor- respond to blasts. It has not been well studied whether this automated five-part differential detects more abnormalities than the Coulter- principle automated differential described above.

A

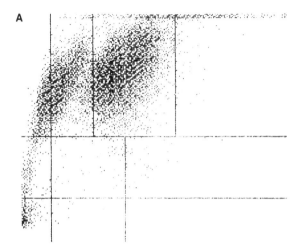

FIGURE 4.12
Cytochemical differential: monocytosis and eosinophilia. (a) Monocytosis. (b) Eosinophilia. Source: Copyright 1983 Technicon Instruments Corporation, Tarrytown, New York.

B

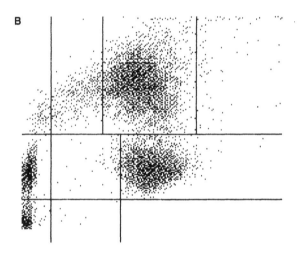

The measurement of myeloperoxidase has allowed the detection of myeloperoxidase abnormalities—either congenital abnormal myeloperoxidase or acquired myeloperoxidase deficiency (Parry et al. 1981; Kitahara et al. 1981; Ross and Bardwell 1980). This is an example of the automated technology allowing new detection of abnormality, in addition to improved precision, speed, or cost.

4.4 Flow Measurements: Light Scatter

The principle of the Ortho flow differential is that different leukocyte types have different size (forward light scatter) and density (90° light scatter). There is a three-part leukocyte differential based on this technology that is under extensive evaluation (Tisdale 1985; J. Koepke, personal communication).

Appendix A
Examples of Abnormal
Automated Blood Counts

Introduction

The best evaluation is made when the history, physical examination, and microscopic review of the blood smear also are included. Definitive diagnosis and management should not be based on the automated count alone. However, the automated count is so often the first available hematologic information that it should be used to best advantage. The examples given below show how the automated count can focus the differential diagnosis to one or a few choices. The history, physical examination, automated count, and blood smear may well indicate the single diagnosis. Some cases will not be so clear-cut. If more than one diagnosis remains possible, the next level of examination can be directed to choose among the few possibilities that are suggested by the initial data, rather than an unfocused, lengthy, and expensive "anemia workup."

Expertise in analyzing the initial data allows many if not most hematologic abnormalities to be detected and classified quickly, leaving more time for the unclear cases. Abnormalities in the automated count will alert the technologist and pathologist to look for corroboration or further abnormalities in the peripheral blood smear, and the clinician, to look for corroboration in the history, physical, and other laboratory data.

Self-Test Cases

The ten unknown cases that follow (figs. A.1–10) illustrate ten common hematologic abnormalities. See what can be deduced from the data (answers are provided in the following section). The peripheral blood smear should always be correlated with the automated data when possible, but the automated count might be all that is initially available. A nomogram of platelet count and MPV in normals is included so the reader can plot the patient data. The routine of analysis should become familiar in the process of working through these test-cases. Although the examples shown are from Coulter instruments, similar analysis is possible with any instrument offering these variables.

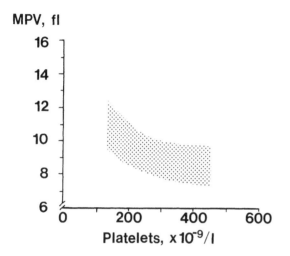

MPV, fl

Platelets, x 10⁻⁹/l

FIGURE A.1

A 49-year-old woman is seen in an oncology clinic for interval treatment of non-Hodgkin's lymphoma.

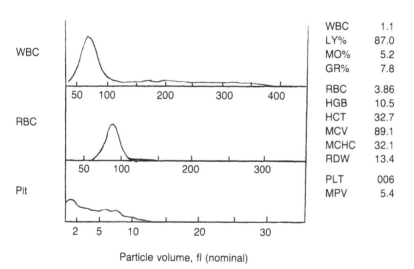

Particle volume, fl (nominal)

WBC	1.1
LY%	87.0
MO%	5.2
GR%	7.8
RBC	3.86
HGB	10.5
HCT	32.7
MCV	89.1
MCHC	32.1
RDW	13.4
PLT	006
MPV	5.4

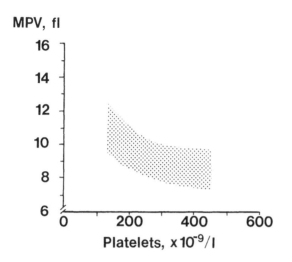

MPV, fl

Platelets, x 10⁻⁹/l

FIGURE A.2

A 54-year-old man is seen in a hematology clinic. He states he has been trans- fused in the past for anemia, but that he now is cured with medicine.

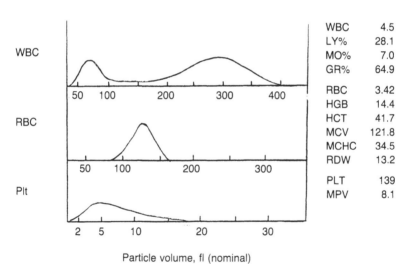

Particle volume, fl (nominal)

WBC	4.5
LY%	28.1
MO%	7.0
GR%	64.9
RBC	3.42
HGB	14.4
HCT	41.7
MCV	121.8
MCHC	34.5
RDW	13.2
PLT	139
MPV	8.1

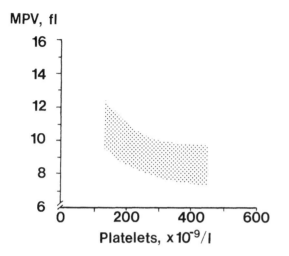

MPV, fl

FIGURE A.3
A 67-year-old man is participating in a senior citizens' blood bank drive.

Platelets, x10⁻⁹/l

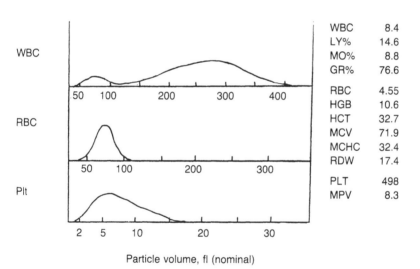

WBC	8.4
LY%	14.6
MO%	8.8
GR%	76.6
RBC	4.55
HGB	10.6
HCT	32.7
MCV	71.9
MCHC	32.4
RDW	17.4
PLT	498
MPV	8.3

Particle volume, fl (nominal)

MPV, fl

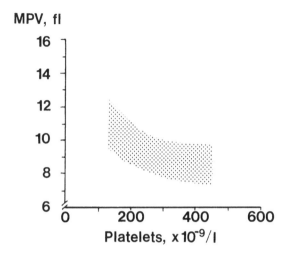

Platelets, x10⁻⁹/l

FIGURE A.4

A 22-year-old medical student is seen in an emergency room for symptoms of pneumonia.

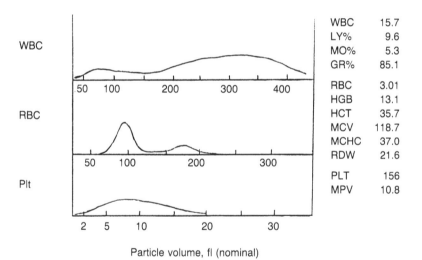

WBC	15.7
LY%	9.6
MO%	5.3
GR%	85.1
RBC	3.01
HGB	13.1
HCT	35.7
MCV	118.7
MCHC	37.0
RDW	21.6
PLT	156
MPV	10.8

Particle volume, fl (nominal)

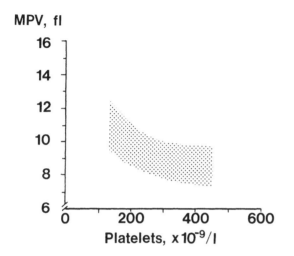

MPV, fl

Platelets, x 10⁻⁹/l

FIGURE A.5

A 46-year-old woman has been referred to a hematology clinic for leukemia.

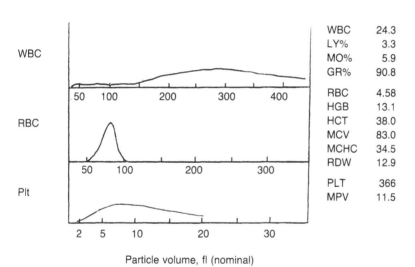

WBC

RBC

Plt

Particle volume, fl (nominal)

WBC	24.3
LY%	3.3
MO%	5.9
GR%	90.8
RBC	4.58
HGB	13.1
HCT	38.0
MCV	83.0
MCHC	34.5
RDW	12.9
PLT	366
MPV	11.5

113

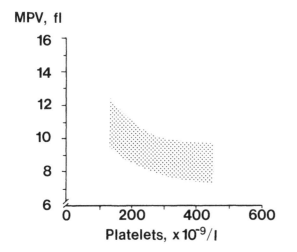

MPV, fl

Platelets, x 10⁻⁹/l

FIGURE A.6
A 24-year-old man is seen in an emergency room for abdominal pain.

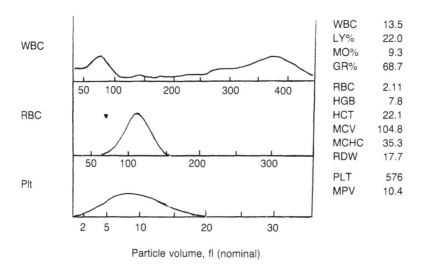

Particle volume, fl (nominal)

WBC	13.5
LY%	22.0
MO%	9.3
GR%	68.7
RBC	2.11
HGB	7.8
HCT	22.1
MCV	104.8
MCHC	35.3
RDW	17.7
PLT	576
MPV	10.4

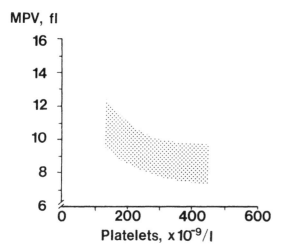

FIGURE A.7
A 26-year-old man has come in to participate in a gay community screening project for detection of acquired immuno-deficiency.

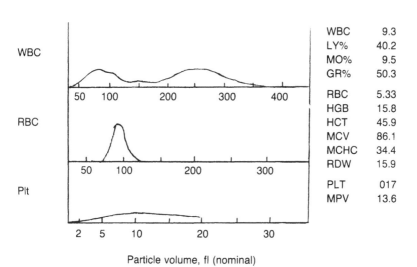

Particle volume, fl (nominal)

WBC	9.3
LY%	40.2
MO%	9.5
GR%	50.3
RBC	5.33
HGB	15.8
HCT	45.9
MCV	86.1
MCHC	34.4
RDW	15.9
PLT	017
MPV	13.6

115

MPV, fl

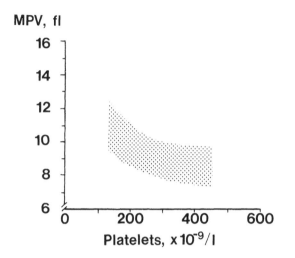

FIGURE A.8
A 54-year-old woman is being seen for a routine interval checkup in a surgical clinic.

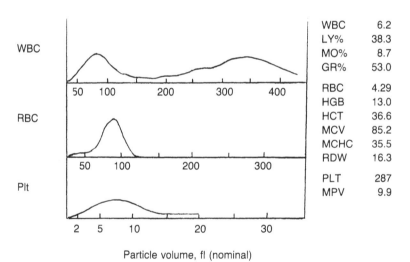

WBC	6.2
LY%	38.3
MO%	8.7
GR%	53.0
RBC	4.29
HGB	13.0
HCT	36.6
MCV	85.2
MCHC	35.5
RDW	16.3
PLT	287
MPV	9.9

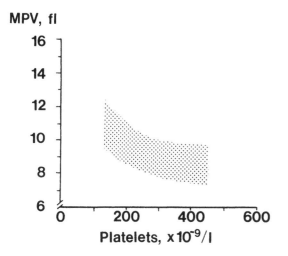

MPV, fl

FIGURE A.9

A 53-year-old man is being evaluated because of cervical lymphade-nopathy.

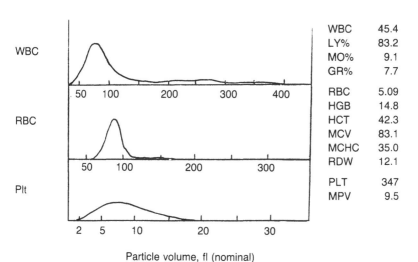

WBC	45.4
LY%	83.2
MO%	9.1
GR%	7.7
RBC	5.09
HGB	14.8
HCT	42.3
MCV	83.1
MCHC	35.0
RDW	12.1
PLT	347
MPV	9.5

Particle volume, fl (nominal)

117

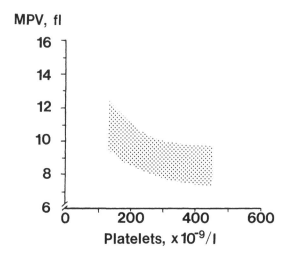

MPV, fl

Platelets, x 10⁻⁹/l

FIGURE A.10

A 37-year-old woman is referred to a clinic for longstanding iron deficiency.

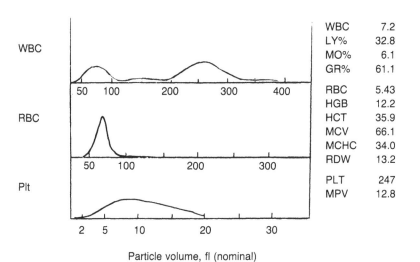

WBC

RBC

Plt

Particle volume, fl (nominal)

WBC	7.2
LY%	32.8
MO%	6.1
GR%	61.1
RBC	5.43
HGB	12.2
HCT	35.9
MCV	66.1
MCHC	34.0
RDW	13.2
PLT	247
MPV	12.8

Answers to Self-Test Cases

Cytotoxic Chemotherapy (fig. A.1)

The white cells are nearly absent, and the histogram shows only lymphocytes. The red cells are reduced in numbers, normocytic (normal MCV), and homogeneous (normal RDW). The platelets are so reduced in number that the count, whether done by slide, phase microscopy, or automated instrument, is only nominal. These data indicate impaired production of all cell lines. Severe sepsis, drug toxicity, megaloblastic anemia, or aplastic anemia could produce pancytopenia. However, this degree of severity is unlikely in the first and third, while the normocytic, homogeneous red cells are against the third and fourth (unless the patient had been extensively transfused). These red cell indices suggest a hypoplastic but not megaloblastic effect of the chemotherapy. In extreme cases, tumor replacement of the bone marrow also may produce the same values.

Aplastic Anemia (fig. A.2)

The cell counts are normal and the white cells are normal in both number and type. Note, however, that other variables are abnormal: the red cells are macrocytic and homogeneous, whereas the platelets are reduced in MPV for the low-normal count. Macrocytic homogeneous anemia has a differential limited essentially to aplastic anemia, preleukemia, and a few cases of early vitamin B_{12} deficiency. The low MPV further suggests one of these three disorders. In contrast, folate deficiency would have a high RDW and, with so high an MCV, would usually, though not always, include anemia. The choice between aplastic anemia, vitamin B_{12} deficiency, and preleukemia cannot be made from the numbers. The history gives the information that allows the final choice. Macrocytosis with normal RDW and hematocrit is typical of "recovery" from aplastic anemia. Vitamin B_{12} deficiency in remission is not macrocytic. Preleukemia is very rarely curable. These results illustrate that a drug-induced remission of aplastic anemia does not abolish the abnormal phenotype of the blood cells but increases their proliferation.

Iron Deficiency (fig. A.3)

The white cells are normal in number and type. The red cells are normal in number, but the MCV is reduced and the RDW elevated (microcytic heterogeneous). The red cell histogram shows no fragments. The platelet count is increased with an MPV within the high-count extrapolation of the nomogram of normals. The red cell pattern is typical only of iron deficiency anemia or, much more rarely, anemic thalassemia (H disease, β-thalassemia intermedia, sickle-thalassemia). Hemoglobin H disease may go undetected into adulthood; the other two rarely do. Note how limited the differential diagnosis is based solely on the red cell findings. Thalassemia trait is excluded by the high RDW. Red cell fragmentation is excluded as a cause of low MCV because no fragments are seen. In extremely severe iron deficiency with markedly low MCV and high RDW, the platelet count, MPV, and MCV all may be affected by small red cells. MCV is altered because the red cells <36 fl are not counted as red cells. For the same reason, the red cell count is falsely low. These artifacts were not seen in this case.

Cold Agglutinins (fig. A.4)

The white cell count is increased because of neutrophilia. Although the hemoglobin is low-normal, the MCV is high, MCHC is high, and the red cell count is low. RDW is markedly increased and the red cell distribution shows one peak with a mode at 93 fl and a second smaller one with a mode at 171 fl. The platelet count and MPV are normal. This set of data is essentially pathognomonic for red cell agglutinins, whether or not they are biologically active in vivo. Neutrophilia has many inflammatory or infectious causes: in this case, pneumonia.

Chronic Myelogenous Leukemia (fig. A.5)

The white cell count is elevated and the differential shows marked neutrophil predominance. However, the distribution of white cells is nearly a single plateau. The red cell count is slightly reduced with normocytic homogeneous indices. The platelets are normal in number but increased in MPV. This abnormal white cell distribution and high MPV together suggest strongly one of two myeloproliferative disorders: chronic myelogenous leukemia or myelofibrosis. In chronic myelogenous leukemia, the RDW may be normal or abnormal; in myelofibrosis, the RDW is abnormally high.

Sickle Cell Anemia (fig. A.6)

The white cell count is slightly increased. In addition to a normal percentage of neutrophils and lymphocytes, there is a shoulder on the small end of the lymphocyte peak—in the nucleated red cell range. Nucleated red cells were 5 per 100 white cells. The MCV is high and the RDW is increased. The platelets are increased and the MPV is large for the count. The macrocytic heterogeneous anemia is consistent with cytotoxic chemotherapy, chronic liver disease, megaloblastic anemia, immune hemolytic anemia, or sickle cell anemia. The thrombocytosis with high MPV is most consistent with sickle cell anemia. Also, nucleated red cells are unusually numerous for the first two.

Immune Thrombocytopenia and Early Iron Deficiency (fig. A.7)

The white cells are normal in number and type. The red cells are normal in number, and are normocytic but heterogeneous; no fragments appear at the left of the peak. The platelets are markedly reduced and MPV is markedly elevated. The high MPV clearly is not caused by red cell fragmentation, and therefore indicates a hyperdestructive platelet disorder or early platelet regeneration after marrow suppression. Despite otherwise normal red cell values, the RDW is high. Particularly in the thrombocytopenic patient, high RDW without other known cause should prompt investigation for early nutritional deficiency. The MCV in the low-normal range suggests iron rather than folate or vitamin B_{12} deficiency.

Red Cell Fragmentation (fig. A.8)

The white cells are normal in number and type. The red cells are slightly reduced in number; MCV is normal, but RDW is increased. Although there are many causes for normocytic heterogeneous anemia, the red cell histogram here points to a single cause. Red cell fragments are visible as a low plateau to the small side of the main peak of cells. The platelet count is normal with a normal MPV. Although some red cell fragments are <20 fl, they are relatively too few to affect substantially the platelet values because the platelet count is normal. These data are consistent with the disease in this patient—excess hemolysis by a prosthetic heart valve.

Chronic Lymphocytic Leukemia (fig. A.9)

The white cells are increased in number, and lymphocytes are predominant, although the granulocyte number is normal. The red cells and platelets are normal in number and size. This is typical of early chronic lymphocytic leukemia.

Heterozygous α-Thalassemia (fig. A.10)

The white cells are normal in number and type. The red cells are normal in number, MCV is low, and RDW is normal. The platelets are normal in number and increased in MPV. Microcytic homogeneous indices may indicate either chronic disease or heterozygous thalassemia. There is no anemia here, so chronic disease cannot be invoked. A normal RDW is very unlikely in iron deficiency. The large platelets are an additional clue (which occurs about 50 percent of the time) to heterozygous thalassemia.

Appendix B
Current Instrumentation

The illustrations shown here provide examples of the data reports of six automated blood counters, manufactured by Coulter, Toa, Sequoia-Turner, Ortho, and Technicon. No endorsement of any particular model is intended. The variables marked with an asterisk have not, to my knowledge, had extensive clinical evaluation or publication concerning clinical use.

Cell-Dyn 200 (Sequoia-Turner, Mountain View, Calif.) (fig. *B.1*)

From top to bottom, the three histograms represent the white cell, red cell, and platelet volume distributions, scaled in femtoliters (fl). At the left are listed: (top) white cell count, and lymphocyte, mid cell* (see note at bottom of illustration), and granulocyte number and percentage; (middle) red cell count, hemoglobin, hematocrit, MCV, MCH, MCHC, and red cell distribution width (RDW*); and (bottom) platelet count. The RDW is calculated as the coefficient of variation. This instrument was offered commercially in late 1985.

Coulter Counter model S-Plus IV
(Coulter, Hialeah, Fla.) (fig. *B.2*)

This data report is typical of the S-Plus series models S-Plus II through S-Plus VI, but not of the model S-Plus. From top to bottom, the three histograms represent the white cell, red cell, and platelet volume distributions, scaled in femtoliters

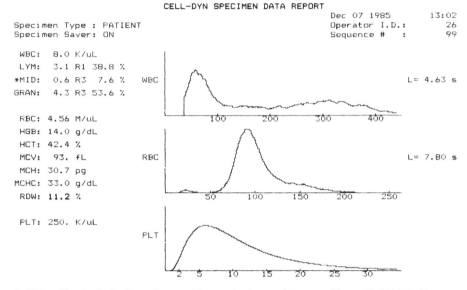

CELL-DYN SPECIMEN DATA REPORT

Dec 07 1985   13:02
Specimen Type : PATIENT   Operator I.D.:   26
Specimen Saver: ON   Sequence # :   99

WBC: 8.0 K/uL
LYM: 3.1 R1 38.8 %
*MID: 0.6 R3 7.6 %   WBC   L= 4.63 s
GRAN: 4.3 R3 53.6 %

RBC: 4.56 M/uL
HGB: 14.0 g/dL
HCT: 42.4 %
MCV: 93. fL   RBC   L= 7.80 s
MCH: 30.7 pg
MCHC: 33.0 g/dL
RDW: 11.2 %

PLT: 250. K/uL
                      PLT

* MID cells include less frequently occurring and rare cells correlating to
monocytes, eosinophils, basophils, blasts and other precursor white cells.

FIGURE B.1
Cell-Dyn 200

(fl). At the right are listed: (top) white cell count, and lymphocyte, monocyte, and granulocyte percentage and number; (middle) red cell count, hemoglobin, hematocrit, MCV, MCH, MCHC, and red cell distribution width (RDW); and (bottom) platelet count, platelet-crit, mean platelet volume (MPV), and platelet distribution width (PDW). The RDW is calculated as the coefficient of variation in these models but not in the S-Plus.

Prototype Coulter automated blood counter
(fig. *B.3*)

At the top left is a distributional scattergram* of the white cell size and cytoplasmic resistance, scaled in arbitrary units, with identified clusters of basophils (BA), eosinophils (EO), lymphocytes (LY), monocytes (MO), and neutrophils (NE). At the bottom left is a nomogram of the normal range of the platelet count, × 10⁹/l, and mean platelet volume (MPV), scaled in femtoliters (fl), against which a specimen's values can be con-

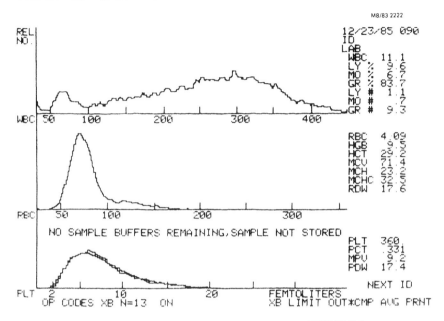

FIGURE B.2
Coulter Counter S-Plus IV

trasted. The histograms at the right are displayed as in figure A. Instead of the granulocyte number, the neutrophil, eosinophil*, and basophil* numbers are given. The platelet-crit and platelet distribution width are omitted. This instrument was not commercially available at the time of publication.

Sysmex E-5000 (Toa, Del Amo, Calif.) (fig. *B.4*)

From top to bottom, the three histograms represent the white cell, red cell, and platelet volume distributions, scaled in femtoliters (fl). At the right are listed: (top) white cell count; (middle) red cell count, hemoglobin, hematocrit, MCV, MCH, MCHC; and (bottom) platelet count. At the bottom right are the percentages of small cells (lymphocytes), middle cells, and large cells (granulocytes). The red cell distribution width is calculated as the standard deviation, as is the platelet distribution width. The mean platelet volume is scaled in fl, and the platelet large cell ratio is the percentage over 12 fl.

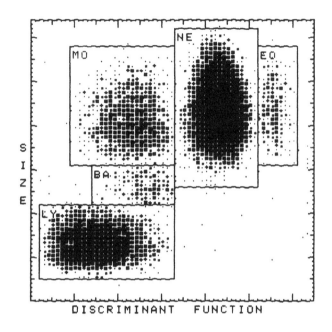

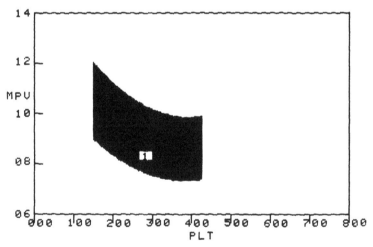

FIGURE B.3
Prototype Coulter counter

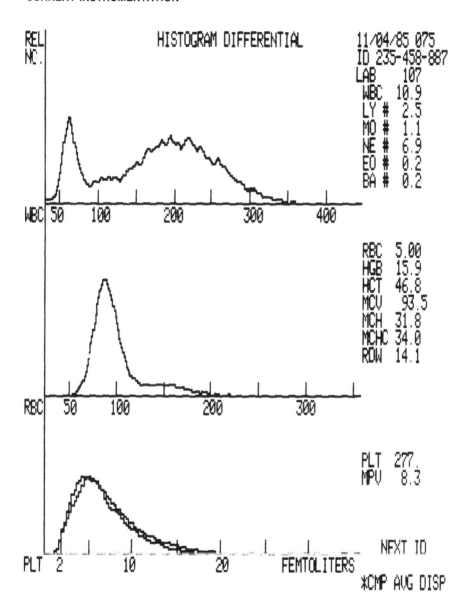

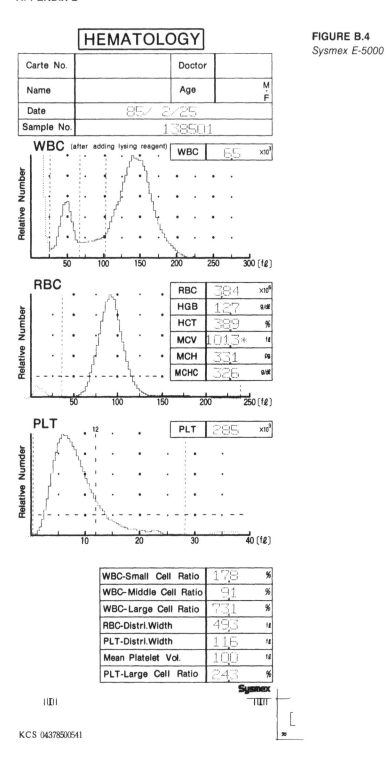

FIGURE B.4
Sysmex E-5000

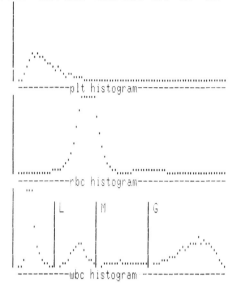

```
       Composite   -- Accession No.000001106  Date  12/07/85
WBC  6.8  RBC 4.75  HGB 14.7  HCT 40.5  MCV  85.  MCH 30.9  MCHC 36.3  PLT 247.
LYM% 24.7  MON% 12.3  GRN% 63.0  LYM  1.7  MON   .8  GRN  4.3  RCMI  -3.7*
```

FIGURE B.5
Ortho ELT-8

Ortho ELT-8 (Ortho, Westwood, Mass.)
(fig. *B.5*)

From top to bottom, the three histograms represent the platelet, red cell, and white cell volume distributions. Across the top are listed: white cell count, red cell count, hemoglobin, hematocrit, MCV, MCH, MCHC, and platelet count; lymphocyte, monocyte, and granulocyte percentage and number; and red cell morphology index (RCMI*).

Technicon H-1 (Technicon, Tarrytown, N.Y.)
(fig. *B.6*)

At the top left are listed: white cell count, red cell count, hemoglobin, hematocrit, MCV, MCH, MCHC, red cell distribution width (RDW), and the coefficient of variation of the red cell hemoglobin (HDW*); platelet count, and mean platelet volume (MPV). The RDW is calculated as the

131

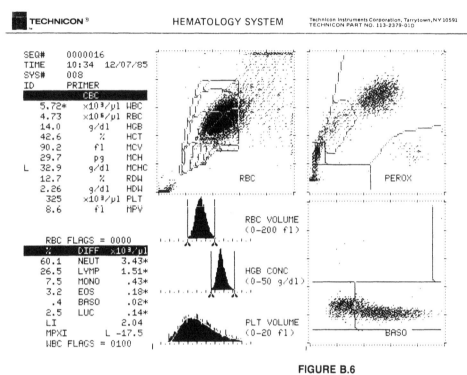

TECHNICON ®

HEMATOLOGY SYSTEM

Technicon Instruments Corporation, Tarrytown, NY 10591
TECHNICON PART NO. 113-2379-01D

```
SEQ#      0000016
TIME      10:34  12/07/85
SYS#      008
ID        PRIMER
          CBC
  5.72*   x10³/µl  WBC
  4.73    x10⁶/µl  RBC
 14.0     g/dl     HGB
 42.6     %        HCT
 90.2     fl       MCV
 29.7     pg       MCH
L 32.9    g/dl     MCHC
 12.7     %        RDW
  2.26    g/dl     HDW
 325      x10³/µl  PLT
  8.6     fl       MPV

   RBC FLAGS = 0000
    %     DIFF   x10³/µl
 60.1   NEUT    3.43*
 26.5   LYMP    1.51*
  7.5   MONO     .43*
  3.2   EOS      .18*
   .4   BASO     .02*
  2.5   LUC      .14*
 LI             2.04
 MPXI        L -17.5
 WBC FLAGS = 0100
```

RBC

PEROX

RBC VOLUME
(0-200 fl)

HGB CONC
(0-50 g/dl)

PLT VOLUME
(0-20 fl)

BASO

FIGURE B.6
Technicon H-1

coefficient of variation. At the bottom left are listed: neutrophil, lymphocyte, monocyte, eosinophil, basophil, and large unstained cells (LUC) percentage and number. The scattergram* at the top middle shows two types of red cell light scatter, from which the standard deviation of the hemoglobin (HDW*) is calculated. At the bottom middle are histograms of the red cell volume, hemoglobin concentration*, and platelet volume distribution. At the right are scattergrams of the several white cell types (basophils at the bottom); the axes are size and peroxidase or alcian blue staining. Lobe index (LI*) is calculated as an assay of granulocyte lobularity. This instrument was offered commercially in late 1985. The Technicon H6000/601C offers these data except for the HDW, hemoglobin scattergram, hemoglobin distribution histogram, and LI.

Glossary

ACD   Acid-citrate dextrose anticoagulant.

Agglutination   Cells sticking together. This may occur with erythrocytes, granulocytes, or platelets.

Anisocytosis   Literally, deviation from similarity among cells. This term is conventionally used to indicate the subjective impression from the peripheral blood smear that the cells vary more than normally in area. It often is graded—slight, moderate, marked; or 1, 2, 3, 4$^+$. Theoretically, anisocytosis is quite different from poikilocytosis (q.v.). In practice the two so often are used as part of a single phrase: for example, "slight aniso- and poikilocytosis." Less commonly used is *anisochromia,* which means the subjective impression from the peripheral smear that the cells vary more than normally in hemoglobin concentration.

Aplastic   See hypoplastic.

CV   *Coefficient of variation.* A standard statistical term to express the relation between absolute variation within the sample (standard deviation, SD) and the mean value of the sample. CV is the SD divided by the mean. Thus, a sample with a mean value of 100 ml and an SD of 1 ml, and a sample with a mean value of 1 ml and an SD of 0.01 ml would have different means and SDs, but the same CV. In each case the variation is 1 percent of the mean value—very little. Obviously, a sample with a mean value of 1 ml and an SD of 1 ml would have a CV of 100 percent. We are used to using CV in quality control—as for example, of pipetting. A 1-ml error in a 1-ml sample would be considered very sloppy pipetting. In contrast, among 100 ml samples, "only 1 ml" variation might be tolerated as acceptable pipetting. The same judgment can be made for the product of repetitive cell divisions as for the product of multiple pipettings: the smaller the CV, the better controlled the process has been.

Cytometry   Literally, measurement of cells. Although this can be accomplished with visual as well as automated methods, increasingly the latter are used.

Diluent   The solution by which blood is diluted in order to produce a cell concentration easily dealt with. Automated counters use various proprietary formulas which are changed periodically.

Dimorphic   Two populations.

Discrete   Separate. In discussing heterogeneity, discrete is used in contrast to nondiscrete. *Discrete* implies there are separate subsets, that are assumed even if they cannot be demonstrated. This is what most discussions of biologic heterogeneity deal with. *Nondiscrete* implies that the variability of the cell property cannot be used to distinguish or infer subsets, but rather is present as a range within a single population. This type of heterogeneity is what is seen in replicate error, quality control, and so forth. I am making a case that any cell characteristic has a degree of nondiscrete heterogeneity, ranging from trivial to enormous, that is part of that cell characteristic's biology. Discreet and its opposite, indiscreet, have rather different meanings.

EDTA   An anticoagulant commonly used for maintaining blood specimens for cell counting ("purple top" tubes). It may be either liquid or powder.

Erythropoiesis   The process of red cell production, primarily in the bone marrow.

Gaussian   A common statistical description of distribution within a population. It assumes the distribution is symmetrical, and has a single peak. Theoretically, it does not reach precisely zero on either end. For red cells, this would mean that in a large enough population there would be a few with subzero volumes. This theoretical assumption has been used to criticize the use of Gaussian statistics to describe red cell size distributions. Because red cell size is the result of influences of cell division, hemoglobin production, membrane formation, red cell deformability, reticulocyle percentage, and red cell aging, it is not surprising that a simple mathematical model will not fit the observed data perfectly. However, the observed data in normal red cell distributions fit a Gaussian distribution so closely that it is appropriate to take advantage of the ease of Gaussian analysis. Gaussian distributions can be described simply by the mean and the standard deviation (see also *log-normal*).

Hematocrit   Originally, the apparatus to determine the percentage of whole blood that was red cells. By extension, the term was then used to describe the percentage value. Finally, the term has been used for automated instruments to describe the product of red cell number times red cell size, per whole blood volume. This resembles, but is not identical to, the second meaning.

Hemoglobinopathy   Abnormality of the amino acid content of the globin portion of the hemoglobin molecule.

Hemolytic Abnormality of red cells in which they are abnormally short-lived, because of accelerated destruction. The cause may be "intrinsic," a defect of some aspect of the red cell itself (e.g., the hemoglobin, a cytoplasmic enzyme, or a membrane protein) or it may be "extrinsic," an abnormally destructive environment for the red cell (e.g., an antibody to the red cell membrane, or a traumatic cardiac valve).

Histogram A display of the frequency distribution of a characteristic among a population. It is a curve in the cell-size display of most instruments.

Hypertonic A solution that has a greater molar concentration of solutes than does normal human plasma or serum. A *hypotonic* solution has a lower molar concentration; an *isotonic* solution, a roughly equal molar concentration.

Hypoproliferative A disorder in which blood cell formation is quantitatively less than normal; also called *hypoplastic.* The extreme case is *aplastic,* in which none of the cell type in question is produced.

Impedance Interruption of electric current. This is the detection principle of "Coulter-type" instruments: the degree to which an electric current is interrupted is directly proportionate to the size (volume) of the object interrupting the current.

Light Scatter Dispersion of a focused light beam by an object in the beam's path. This is the detection principle of certain automated instruments: the degree to which the beam is dispersed is directly proportional to the size (volume) of the object dispersing the beam.

Log-Normal Distribution of a property such that it is symmetrical if the ordinate is in a logarithmic scale, and right-skewed if the ordinate is in an arithmetic scale. Theoretically, a log-normal distribution includes cells infinitely large, though not subzero. Thus, as a model the log-normal distribution is as theoretically imperfect as the Gaussian. Practically, platelet and leukocyte histograms are right-skewed and similar enough to log-normal distributions to make log-normal analysis appropriate.

Macrocytic See *Normocytic.*

MCH Mean cell hemoglobin.

MCHC Mean cell hemoglobin concentration.

MCV Mean cell volume.

Microcytic See *Normocytic.*

Morphology Literally, the study of form. "Classical" morphology is the description of size, shape, color, and so forth by light microscopy. However, form measured by electron microscopy or flow cytometry also can be considered morphology.

MPV Mean platelet volume.

Myelofibrosis See *Myelophthisic.*

Myelophthisic Literally, consumption of marrow. This describes conditions in which the marrow is replaced by something else—tumor, granuloma, or fibrous tissue (the latter is called *myelofibrosis*). Normal marrow cell production then is progressively reduced in amount, giving a *hypoproliferative* (q.v.) picture. However, often the marrow also prematurely releases cells, that is, young reticulocytes, nucleated red cells, and myelocytes, the classical "myelophthistic" peripheral blood abnormalities.

Myeloproliferative Abnormal, generally increased marrow production. By convention this generally does not refer to acute leukemias, nor to hemoglobinopathies, but rather to chronic myelogenous leukemia, polycythemia vera, essential thrombocytosis, and refractory anemia with excess blasts. The marrow has an increased cellularity, but this is not necessarily paralleled by increased peripheral blood counts. Rather, there may be ineffective marrow cell maturation, so that cells die or are destroyed before they reach the peripheral blood. An overlapping term is *myelodysplastic.*

Normocytic Normal size. *Microcytic* means less-than-normal size; *macrocytic,* greater than normal.

PDW Platelet distribution width.

Ploidy The amount of DNA in a cell (generally, in the cell nucleus). Most cells are diploid, which by convention is denoted 2c or 2n. Diploid cells in mitosis progressively increase their DNA content to 4n, and then mitosis produces two cells, each with 2n DNA. Megakaryocytes are thought to have nuclear replication without cell division, and so have DNA content in several progressive powers of 2: 2n, 4n, 8n, 16n, 32n, 64n, 128n. Osteoclasts also have various multiple-of-2 amounts of DNA: 2n, 4n, 6n, 8n, 10n. Plasma cells (and hepatocytes) also may be multinuclear and so have 2n, 4n, or 6n DNA. All of these cell types in which the nonmitotic DNA content is 4n or greater are called *polyploid.*

Poikilocytosis Variability of cell shape. This, strictly speaking, is independent of size, and refers to target cells, spherocytes, sickle cells, fragments, and so forth. In practice, size and shape are assessed together in light microscopic examination (see also *Anisocytosis*).

RDW Red cell distribution width.

Reticulocyte The stage of red cell maturation after the nucleus is extended. Residual RNA is still present in the cytoplasm. Cells with sufficient RNA have a more bluish tinge than those red cells without RNA, when stained with the usual Wright's preparation. Such cells are described as "polychromatophilic." The more quantitative descriptor is presence of RNA by a supravital stain specific for RNA—classically, new methylene blue. Other stains, such as acridine orange and phycoerythrin, also are being tried. Because RNA remains in red cells for only one to two days after their entry into peripheral blood, reticulocyte number indicates the amount of red cell production. Reticulocyte percentage indicates the proportion of cells newly produced; in the steady state this suggests whether the red cell life span is shortened or not.

Thalassemia Literally, a blood disorder from the Mediterranean. This group of disorders first was described in Mediterraneans, but, in fact, is found worldwide among populations historically exposed to malaria. The thalassemias are disorders in which the globin chains are structurally correct. However, because of abnormal DNA structure and/or RNA processing, the chains intracellularly are quantitatively imbalanced because of hypoproduction of either the α or the non-α chain (see text).

References

Akwari AM, Ross DW, Stass SA. Spuriously elevated platelet counts due to microspherocytosis. Am J Clin Path 1982; 77:220–1.

Armitage JD, Goeken JA, Feagler JR. Spurious elevation of the platelet count in acute leukemia. JAMA 1978; 239:433–4.

Bates JM, Bessman JD. Red cell precursors in aplastic anemia are macrocytic before hemoglobin formation. Clin Res 1986; (abstract) 34:216a.

Bator JM, Groves MR, Price BJ, Eckstein FC. Erythrocytic deformability and size measured in a multi-parameter system that includes impedance sizing. Cytometry 1984; 5:34–41.

Baynes RD, Flax H, Bothwell TH, et al. Red blood cell distribution width in the anemia secondary to tuberculosis. Am J Clin Path 1986; 85:226–9.

Beautyman W, Bills T. Osmotic error in erythrocyte volume determinations. Am J Hem 1982; 12:383–9.

Bessman JD. Erythropoiesis during recovery from iron deficiency: normocytes and macrocytes. Blood 1977a; 50:987–94.

Bessman JD. Erythropoiesis during recovery from macrocytic anemia: macrocytes, normocytes, and microcytes. Blood 1977b; 48:995–1000.

Bessman JD. Microcytosis caused by red cell fragmentation. JAMA 1977c; 238:2391–2.

Bessman JD. Heterogeneity of human red cell volume. Quantitation, clinical correlation, and possible mechanisms. Johns Hopkins Med J 1980a; 146:228–32.

Bessman JD. Spurious macrocytosis: a common clue to erythrocyte cold agglutinins. Am J Clin Path 1980b; 74:797–800.

Bessman JD. Prediction of platelet production during recovery from acute leukemia. Am J Hem 1982; 13:219–27.

Bessman JD. The relation of megakaryocyte ploidy to platelet size. Am J Hem 1984; 16:161–70.

Bessman JD. Use of mean platelet volume improves detection of platelet disorders. Blood Cells 1985; 11:127–36.

REFERENCES

Bessman JD. Reticulocytes. In: Hurst JW and Hall GD, eds. Clinical medicine, 3rd edition. 1986 (in press).

Bessman JD, Dover GJ. Distribution of erythrocyte volume during the transition from fetal to adult erythropoiesis. Blood 1978; 52:76a (abstract).

Bessman JD, Feinstein DI. Quantitative anisocytosis as a discriminant between iron deficiency and thalassemia minor. Blood 1979; 53:288–93.

Bessman JD, Gardner FH. Platelet size in thrombocytopenia due to sepsis. Surg Gyn Obst 1983; 156:177–80.

Bessman JD, Gardner FH. Persistence of abnormal red cell and platelet phenotype during recovery from aplastic anemia. Arch Int Med 1985; 145:293–6.

Bessman JD, Gilmer PR, Gardner FH. Improved classification of anemia by MCV and RDW. Am J Clin Path 1983; 80:332–6.

Bessman JD, Hurley EW, Groves MR. Nondiscrete heterogeneity of human erythrocytes: comparison of Coulter-principle flow cytometry and Soret-hemoglobinometry image analysis. Cytometry 1983; 3:292–5.

Bessman JD, Williams LJ, Gilmer PR. Mean platelet volume. Am J Clin Path 1981; 76:289–93.

Bessman JD, Williams LJ, Gilmer PR. Platelet size in health and hematologic disease. Am J Clin Path 1982; 78:150–3.

Bloom GE, Diamond LK. Prognostic value of fetal hemoglobin levels in acquired aplastic anemia. N Eng J Med 1968; 278:304–8.

Brittin GM, Brecher G, Johnson CA, Stuart J. Spurious macrocytosis of antibody-coated red cells. Am J Clin Path 1969; 52:237–40.

Bull BS, Hay KL. Are red blood cell indexes international? Arch Path Lab Med 1985; 109:604–6

Bull BS, Zucker MV. Changes in platelet volume produced by temperature, metabolic inhibitors, and aggregating agents. Proc Soc Exp Biol Med 1965; 120:296–301.

Bunn HF, Forget B. Human hemoglobins, 2nd edition. Philadelphia: Saunders, 1985.

Cameron HA, Phillips R, Ibbotson RM, Carson PHM. Platelet size in myocardial infarction. Brit Med J 1983; 287:449–51.

Camitta BM, Storb R, Thomas ED. Aplastic anemia. N Eng J Med 1982; 306:712–8.

Carmel R, Denson AA, Mussell B. Anemia: textbook versus practice. JAMA 1979; 242:2295–7.

Castro OL, Haddy TB, Rana SR, Worrell KD, Scott RB. Electronically determined red blood cell values in a large number of healthy black adults. Am J Epidem 1985; 121:930–6.

Chalmers DM, Levi AJ, Chanarin I, et al. Mean cell volume in a working population: the effects of age, smoking, alcohol, and oral contraception. Brit J Haem 1979; 43:631–6.

Champlin R, Ho W, Gale RP. Antithymocyte globulin treatment in patients with aplastic anemia: a prospective randomized trial. N Eng J Med 1983; 308:113–8.

Clarkson DS, Moore EM. Reticulocyte size in nutritional anemia. Blood 1976; 48:669–77.

Cornbleet J. Spurious results from automated hematology cell counters. Lab Med 1983; 14:509–14.

Cornbleet PJ, Kessinger S. Accuracy of 1,000 platelet counts on the Coulter S-Plus V. Am J Clin Path 1985; 83:78–80.

Couch JY, Kaplow LS. Relation of reticulocyte age to polychromasia, shift cells, and shift reticulocytes. Arch Path Lab Med 1985; 109:325–30.

Cox CJ, Habermann TJ, Payne PA, Klee GG, Pierre RV. Evaluation of the Coulter Counter model S-Plus IV. Am J Clin Path 1985; 84:297–306.

Davidson RU, Cumming AM, Leel VH, et al. A search for the mechanism underlying the altered MCV in thyroid dysfunction: a study of serum and red cell membrane lipids. Scand J Haem 1984; 32:19–24.

Dighiero G, Lesly C, Lepourier M, Conty MC. Computer analysis of platelet volumes. In: Ross DW, Brecher G, and Bessis M, eds. Automation in hematology. New York: Springer-Verlag, 1981:331–7.

Dover GJ, Ogawa M. Cellular mechanisms for increased fetal hemoglobin products in culture. J Clin Invest 1980; 66:1175–8.

Dutcher TF. Automated leukocyte differentials: a review and prospective. Lab Hem 1983; 14:483–7.

Dutcher TF. Automated differentials: a strategy. Blood Cells 1985; 11:49–60.

Dzik WH. Platelet size in megaloblastic anemia. Am J Clin Path 1982; 79:274 (letter).

Ebbe S, Stohlman F, Overcash LJ, Donovan J, Howard D. Megakaryocyte size in thrombocytopenic and normal rats. Blood 1968; 32:383–91.

Eldor A, Avitzour M, Or R. Prediction of haemorrhagic diathesis in thrombocytopenia by mean platelet volume. Brit Med J 1982; 285:397–400.

Embury SH, Dozy AM, Miller J, et al. Concurrent sickle cell anemia and α-thalassemia: effect on severity of anemia. N Eng J Med 1982; 306:270–4.

England JM. Blood cell sizing. In: Koepke JC, ed. Laboratory hematology. New York: Churchill Livingston, 1984: 927–72.

England JM, Chetty MC, DeSilva PM. Estimation of lymphocyte percentage and number on the Coulter Counter Model S-Plus Phase II. J Clin Path 1982; 34:1194–9.

REFERENCES

England JM, Down MC. Red cell volume distribution curves and the measurement of anisocytosis. Lancet 1974; 1:701–3.

England JM, Fraser P. Discrimination between iron-deficiency and heterozygous thalassaemia syndromes in differential diagnosis of microcytosis. Lancet 1979; 1:145–8.

Epstein CJ, Sahud MA, Piel CF, et al. Hereditary macrothrombocytopathia, nephritis, and deafness. Am J Med 1972; 52:299–310.

Fairbanks VF, Beutler E. Iron deficiency. In: Williams WC, et al., eds. Hematology, 3rd edition. New York: McGraw-Hill, 1983:466–8.

Fay RA, Hughes AG, Farron NT. Platelet hyperdestruction in pregnancy. Obst Gyn 1983; 61:238–40.

Finch CA. Review: erythropoiesis, erythropoietin, and iron. Blood 1982; 59:1241–6.

Freedman ML, Karpatkin S. Elevated platelet count and megathrombocyte count in sickle cell anemia. Blood 1975; 45:579–81.

Friedhoff AJ, Miller, JC, Karpatkin S. Heterogeneity of human platelets VII. Platelet monoamine oxidase activity in normals and patients with autoimmune thrombocytopenic purpura and reactive thrombocytosis: its relation to platelet protein density. Blood 1978; 51:317–23.

Gardner FH, Bessman JD. Thrombocytopenia due to defective platelet production. Clin Haem 1983; 12:33–8.

Garg SK, Amorosi EL, Karpatkin S. Use of the megathrombocyte as an index of megakaryocyte number. N Eng J Med 1971; 184:11–7.

Garg SK, Lackner H, Karpatkin S. The increased percentage of megathrombocytes in various clinical disorders. Ann Int Med 1972; 77:361–9.

Giles C. Intravascular coagulation in gestational hypertension and pre-eclampsia: the value of haematological screening tests. Clin Lab Haem 1982; 4:351–8.

Giles C. The platelet count and mean platelet volume. Brit J Haem 1981; 48:31–8.

Giles C, Inglis TCM. Thrombocytopenia and macrothrombocytosis in gestational hypertension. Brit J Obs Gyn 1981; 88:1115–20.

Gilmer PR, Koepke JA. The reticulocyte: an approach to definition. Am J Clin Path 1976; 66:262–7.

Gilmer PR, Williams LJ, Bessman JD. Spuriously elevated platelet counts due to microspherocytosis. Am J Clin Path 1982; 78:259 (letter).

Gottfried EL. Erythrocyte indexes with the electronic counter. N Eng J Med 1979; 300:1277.

Gralnick HR, Williams SB, Shafer BV, Corash L. Factor VIII/Von

Willebrand factor binding to von Willebrand's disease platelets. Blood 1982; 60:328–32.

Green R, Kulh W, Jacobson R, et al. Masking of macrocytosis by α-thalassemia in blacks with pernicious anemia. N Eng J Med 1982; 307:1322–5.

Hammersley MW, King BW, Sillivant RE, Liu PL, Teaford MJ, Crook L, Biondo CD. High erythrocyte distribution values and possibilities of hemoglobinopathies. Am J Clin Path 1981; 75:370–2.

Hanker JJ, Giammara BL. Neutrophil pseudoplatelets: their discrimination by myeloperoxidase determination. Science 1983; 220:415–7.

Hansen AC, Stahl M. Lymphocyte counting by cell size distribution analysis of leukocytes compared with conventional blood film differential count. Scand J Clin Lab Inv 1984; 44:211–5.

Hansen RM, Hanson C, Anderson T. Failure to suspect and diagnose thalassemic syndromes. Arch Int Med 1985; 145:93–4.

Hattersley PG, Gerard PW, Caggiano V, Nash DR. Erroneous values on the model S Coulter due to high titer cold agglutinins. Am J Clin Path 1971; 55:442–3.

Higgs DR, Aldridge BE, Lamb J, et al. The interaction of alpha thalassemia and sickle cell disease. N Eng J Med 1982; 306:1441–6.

Hillman RS, Finch CA. The misused reticulocyte. Brit J Haem 1969; 17:313–5.

Holme S, Simmonds M, Ballek T, et al. Comparative measurements of platelet size by Coulter counter microscopy of blood smears, and light transmission studies. J Lab Clin Med 1982; 97:610–22.

Howard MA, Hutton RA, Hardisty RM. Hereditary giant platelet syndrome: a disorder of a new aspect of platelet function. Brit Med J 1981; 2:586–8.

Jen P, Woo B, Rosenthal PE, Bunn HF, Loscalzo A, Goldman L. Value of the peripheral blood smear in anemic patients. Arch Int Med 1983; 143:1120–5.

Johnson CS, Moyes D, Schroeder WA, Shelton JR, Beutler E. Hb Pasadena. Identification by high performance liquid chromatography of a new unstable variant with increased oxygen affinity. Biochem Biophys Acta 1980; 223:360–7.

Johnson CS, Tegos C, Beutler E. α-Thalassemia: prevalence and hematologic findings in American blacks. Arch Int Med 1982; 143:1280–1.

Johnson CS, Tegos C, Beutler E. Thalassemia minor: routine erythrocyte measurements and differentiation from iron deficiency. Am J Clin Path 1983; 80:31–6.

REFERENCES

Karpatkin S. Heterogeneity of human platelets VI. Correlation of platelet function with platelet volume. Blood 1978; 51:307–16.

Karpatkin S, Freedman ML. Hypersplenic thrombocytopenia differentiated from increased peripheral platelet destruction by platelet volume. Ann Int Med 1978; 89:200–3.

Karpatkin S, Garg SK, Freedman M. Role of iron as a regulator of thrombopoiesis. Am J Med 1974; 57:521–4.

Kaye FJ, Alter BP. Red cell size distribution analysis: an evaluation of microcytic anemia in chronically ill patients. Mt Sinai J Med 1985; 52:519–23.

Kelly A, Munan L. Haemotologic profile of natural populations: red cell parameters. Brit J Haem 1977; 35:153–60.

Kitahara M, Eyre HJ, Simonian Y, Atkin CI, Hasstedt JJ. Hereditary myeloperoxidase deficiency. Blood 1981; 57:888–93.

Koepke JA, ed. Differential leukocyte counting. Chicago: C.A.P., 1978.

Koepke JA, ed. The white blood cell differential. I. Blood Cells 1985; 11:1–150.

Levin J, Bessman JD. The inverse relationship between platelet volume and platelet number. J Lab Clin Med 1983; 101:295–307.

Levin J, Conley CL. Thrombocytosis associated with malignant disease. Arch Int Med 1964; 114:497–500.

Levine RF, Hazzard KC, Lamberg JD. The significance of megakaryocyte size. Blood 1982; 60:1122–31.

Lippi U, Cappelletti P. Quality control of mean platelet volume: a chimera? Am J Clin Path 1983; 79:648–9 (letter).

Lipschitz DA, Mitchell CO, Thompson C. The anemia of senescence. Am J Hem 1981; 11:47–54.

Lum LG, Tubergen DC, Corash L, Blaese RM. Splenectomy in the management of the thrombocytopenia of the Wiskott-Aldrich syndrome. N Eng J Med 1980; 302:892–6.

McClure S, Custer E, Bessman JD. Improved detection of early iron deficiency by abnormal RDW. JAMA 1985; 253:1021–3.

McDonald ME, Smyrk TC, Payne BA, Pierre RV. Evaluation of the concept of the classification of anemias by use of the RDW/MCV. Blood 1984; 64:45a (abstract).

Mayer K. Presence of abnormal cells. Blood Cells 1985; 11:25–29.

Mayer K, Chin B, Baisley A. Evaluation of the S-Plus IV. Am J Clin Path 1985; 83:40–6.

Meyers LD, Habicht J-P, Johnson CL. Components of the difference in hemoglobin concentrations in blood between black and white women in the United States. Am J Epidem 1979; 109:539–49.

Mezzano D, Hoang K, Catalano P, Aster RH. Evidence that platelet buoyant density, but not size, correlates with platelet age in man. Am J Hem 1981; 11:61–71.

Mundschenk DD, Connelly DP, White JG, Brunning RD. An improved technique for the electronic measurement of platelet size and shape. J Lab Clin Med 1976; 88:301–10.

Murphy S, Oski FA, Naiman JL, Lusch CJ, Goldberg S, Gardner FH. Platelet size and kinetics in hereditary and acquired thrombocytopenia. N Eng J Med 1972; 286:499–504.

Natta C, Weiner MA, Chang H, et al. Sickle cell anemia and iron deficiency: resemblance to sickle thalassemia. JAMA 1982; 247:1442–3.

Nelson, L, Charache S, Keyser E, Metzger P. Laboratory evaluation of the Coulter "three-part electronic differential." Am J Clin Path 1985; 83:547–54.

O'Hare JA, Murnaghan DJ. Reversal of aluminum-induced hemodialysis anemia by a low-aluminum dialysate. N Eng J Med 1982; 306:654–6.

Parry MF, Root RK, Metcalf JA, et al. Myeloperoxidase deficiency: prevalence and clinical significance. Ann Int Med 1981; 95:293–301.

Patel A, Chanarin I. Restoration of normal red cell size after treatment in megaloblastic anaemia. Brit J Haem 1975; 30:57–63.

Paulus JM. Recent advances in the study of megakaryocyte physiology. Pathol Biol 1981; 29:133–5.

Paulus JM, Bury J, Grosdent JC. Control of platelet territory development in megakaryocytes. Blood Cells 1979; 5:59–69.

Paulus JM, Prenant JM, Deschamps JF, et al. Polyploid megakaryocytes develop randomly from a multicompartmental system of committed precursors. Proc Nat Acad Sci 1982; 79:4410–4.

Payne BA, Pierre RV. Pseudothrombocytopenia: A laboratory artifact with potentially serious consequences. Mayo Clin Proc 1984; 59:123–5.

Penington DG, Streatfield K, Roxburgh AE. Megakaryocytes and the heterogeneity of circulating platelets. Brit J Haem 1976; 34:639–53.

Perrotta AL, Finch CA. The polychromatophlic erythrocyte. Am J Clin Path 1972; 57:471–7.

Petrucci JV, Dunne PA, Chapman CC. Spurious erythrocyte indices as measured by the model S Coulter Counter due to cold agglutinins. Am J Clin Path 1971; 56:500–2.

Pierre RV. The automated blood count. American Society of Clinical Pathology Teleconferences, 1984.

Pierre RV. The routine differential leukocyte count vs automated differential counts. Blood Cells 1985; 11:11–24.

Powars DR, Schroeder WA, Weiss JN, et al. Lack of influence of fetal hemoglobin levels or erythrocyte indices on severity of sickle cell anemia. J Clin Invest 1980; 65:732–40.

REFERENCES

Price-Jones C. Red blood cell diameters. Oxford: Oxford University Press, 1922.

Pruzanski W, Shumak H. Biologic activity of cold-reacting antibodies. N Eng J Med 1977; 296:1490–4.

Rappeport JM, Nathan DG. Acquired aplastic anemias: pathophysiology and treatment. Adv Int Med 1982; 27:547–90.

Rich EC, Crowson TW, Connelly DP. Effectiveness of differential leukocyte count in case finding in the ambulatory care setting. JAMA 1983; 249:633–6.

Robbins G, Barnard DL. Thrombocytosis and microthrombocytosis: a clinical evaluation of 371 cases. Acta Haem 1983; 70:175–82.

Rock WA, Grogan JE. Demand versus need versus physician prerogatives in the use of the WBC differential. JAMA 1983; 249:613–6.

Roper PR, Johnston D, Austin J, Agarwal SS, Drewinko B. Profiles of platelet volume distribution in normal individuals and in patients with acute leukemia. Am J Clin Path 1977; 68:449–57.

Ross DW, Bardwell A. Automated cytochemistry and the white cell differential in leukemia. Blood Cells 1980; 6:455–70.

Rowan RM, Fraser C. Platelet size distribution analysis. In: van Assendelft OW and England JM, eds. Advances in haematological methods: the blood count. Boca Raton: CRC Press, 1982:125–42.

Rumke CL, Bezemer PD, Kuik DJ. Normal values and least significant differences for differential leukocyte counts. J Chron Dis 1975; 78:662–8.

Sahud MA. Platelet size and number in alcoholic thrombocytopenia. N Eng J Med 1972; 286:355–6.

Savage RA. An intralaboratory evaluation of the Coulter SII lymphocyte percent as indicative of actual lymphocyte numbers in blood. Am J Clin Path 1985; 83:34–9.

Savage RA, Hoffman GC. Clinical significance of osmotic matrix errors in automated hematology. Am J Clin Path 1983; 80:861–5.

Serjeant GR, Foster K, Serjeant BE. Red cell size and the clinical and haematological features of homozygous sickle cell disease. Brit J Haem 1981; 48:445–9.

Sewell R, Ibbotson RM, Phillips R, Carson P. High mean platelet volume after myocardial infarction: is it due to consumption of small platelets? Brit Med J 1984; 289:1576–9.

Shapiro MF, Hatch RL, Greenfield S. Cost containment and labor intensive tests. The case of the leukocyte differential count. JAMA 1984; 252:231–4.

Shreiner DP, Bell WR. Pseudothrombocytopenia: manifestation of a new type of platelet agglutinin. Blood 1973; 42:541–9.

REFERENCES

Shulman NR, Leissinger CA, Hotchiss AJ, Kauk CA. Platelet debris containing non-specifically absorbed IgG and other membrane markers in an index of platelet destruction. Circulation 1982; 66 (suppl):297 (abstract).

Small BM, Bettigole RE. Diagnosis of myeloproliferative disease by analysis of the platelet volume distribution. Am J Clin Path 1981; 76:685–91.

Solanki DL, Blackburn BC. Spurious red blood cell parameters due to serum cold agglutinins: Observations on the Ortho ELT-8 Cell Counter. Am J Clin Path 1985; 83:218–22.

Spivak JL. Masked megaloblastic anemia. Arch Int Med 1982; 142:2111–4.

Stein J, ed. Internal medicine. Boston: Little Brown, 1983.

Steinberg MH, Adams JH. Thalassemic hemoglobinopathies. Am J Path 1983; 113:396–409.

Steinberg MH, Coleman MB, Adams JG, Rosenstock W. Interaction between HbS and β-thalassemia and α-thalassemia. Clin Res 1984; 31:875a (abstract).

Stoll DB, Blum S, Pasquale D, Murphy S. Thrombocytopenia with decreased megakaryocytes. Ann Int Med 1981; 94:120–75.

Tavassoli M. Megakaryocyte-platelet axis and the process of platelet formation and release. Blood 1980; 55:537–42.

Thomspon CB, Diaz DD, Quinn PG, Lapins M, Kurtz SR, Valeri CR. The role of anticoagulation in the measurement of platelet volumes. Am J Clin Path 1983a; 80:327–32.

Thompson CB, Jakubowski JA, Quinn PG, et al. Platelet size as a determinant of platelet function. J Lab Clin Med 1983b; 101:205–13.

Thompson CB, Love DG, Quinn PG, Valeri CR. Platelet size does not correlate with platelet age. Blood 1983c; 62:487–94.

Threatte GA, Adrados C, Ebbe S, Brecher G. Mean platelet volume: the need for a reference method. Am J Clin Path 1984; 81:769–72.

Tisdale PA. Evaluation of a laser-based three-part leukocyte differential analyzer in detection of clinical abnormalities. Lab Med 1985; 16:228–33.

Trapp GA. Plasma aluminum is bound to transferrin. Life Sci 1983; 33:311–6.

Vainchenker W, Guichard J, Breton-Gorius J. Growth of human megakaryocyte colonies in culture from fetal, neonatal, and adult peripheral blood cells; ultrastructural analysis. Blood Cells 1979; 5:25–37.

van Assendelft OW, England JM. Advances in haematologic methods. Calibration and control. Boca Raton: CRC Press, 1982.

REFERENCES

Van der Lelie J, Brakenhoff JAC. Mean platelet volume in myocardial infarction. Brit Med J 1983; 287:1471 (letter).

Ward PCJ. The new indices. American Society of Clinical Pathology program workshop, 1985.

Weiss GB, Bessman JD. Spurious automated red cell values in warm autoimmune hemolytic anemia. Am J Hem 1984; 17:433–6.

White JG. Ultrastructural studies of the grey platelet syndrome. Am J Path 1979; 95:445–54.

Williams WJ, et al., eds. Hematology, 3rd edition. New York: McGraw-Hill, 1983.

Wintrobe MM. Clinical hematology, 8th edition. Philadelphia: Lea and Febiger, 1981.

Ziegler Z, Murphy S, Gardner FH. Microscopic platelet size and morphology in various hematologic disorders. Blood 1978; 51:479–86.

Zucker-Franklin D, Karpatkin S. Red cell and platelet fragmentation in idiopathic autoimmune thrombocytopenic purpura. N Eng J Med 1977; 297:517–23.

Index

INDEX

Lightning Source UK Ltd.
Milton Keynes UK
UKHW012206170820
368379UK00001B/43